CODE BLUE

CODE BLUE
Reviving Canada's Health Care System

David Gratzer

ECW PRESS

The publication of *Code Blue* has been generously supported by
The Canada Council, the Ontario Arts Council, and by
the Government of Canada through
the Book Publishing Industry Development Program.

CANADIAN CATALOGUING IN PUBLICATION DATA

Gratzer, David
Code blue: reviving Canada's health care system

ISBN 1-55022-393-3

1. Medical care – Canada.
2. National health insurance – Canada.
I. Title.

RA395.C3G72 1999   362.1'0971   C99-931995-7

Printed by AGMV l'Imprimeur, Cap-Saint-Ignace, Quebec.

Distributed by General Distribution Services,
325 Humber College Blvd., Etobicoke, Ontario M9W 7C3.

Published by ECW Press,
2120 Queen Street East, Suite 200,
Toronto, Ontario M4E 1E2.

www.ecw.ca/press

PRINTED AND BOUND IN CANADA

To my family:
George and Catherine,
Tom and Adeena,
Daniel and Anna

Table of Contents

Acknowledgements

While the cover bears only one name, many people helped to turn the idea of a sensible book on health care into a reality.

I owe great thanks to my father for patiently listening to my ideas and offering his own. Every page of this book has benefited from his advice. He served numerous roles in this effort: editor, critic, supporter, and psychotherapist — all without a nickel of compensation.

Code Blue wouldn't have been possible without the encouragement and patience of David Frum and Adrienne Snow. Both had confidence that I could write a book long before I did. One of the great joys of taking on this project was getting to know David and Adrienne better. They are two of the finest people I have ever met.

Terry Corcoran, William Watson, Cynthia Ramsay, Stephen Harper, David Henderson, and Arnold Aberman all read early versions of the manuscript and provided valuable suggestions. Ramsay, in particular, was helpful not simply in sorting out my thoughts but also in assisting my understanding of health economics.

I am grateful to John R. MacKenzie and the Marigold Foundation.

Dallas Harrison did a superlative job editing the manuscript. Robert Lecker, my publisher, took a chance on a young writer, and I am most grateful.

Numerous physicians, administrators, economists, and political staff answered my many questions. Some are quoted herein, while others are not.

I appreciated the encouragement of Marvin Levant and William Goodman, two doctors who began writing sensibly on this topic long ago.

Of course, the responsibility for any mistakes contained in this volume rests with me.

Introduction

ARLY IN 1999, the surgery of a 46-year-old man was cancelled. Such an event isn't unusual in any health care system, but this was no ordinary operation. Daniel Smith suffers from cystic fibrosis. February 3 was the day he was to receive two donated lungs, an urgently needed transplant that could literally breathe new life into his body.

But it didn't work out that way. It wasn't that lungs couldn't be found for the surgery (miraculously, they were) or that the procedure was too difficult or dangerous for doctors to perform. Administrators cancelled the double-lung transplant because no ICU bed could be found for the patient.

Modern medicine wasn't the problem. Medicare was.

It would be easy to dismiss this example as an exception — a tragic and unacceptable shortcoming, but an isolated example. Except that, while Smith was losing his opportunity for life-saving surgery, patients across Canada were having problems getting proper medical care. Here are other examples from February 1999:

- The Ontario government was desperately trying to arrange medical treatment for cancer patients — in the United States. And with good reason. Waiting times far exceeded the clinically recommended four-week period between diagnosis and the start of radiation therapy.
- Emergency rooms were severely overcrowded for a second year in a row, not only in Ontario but also across Canada. At Cité de la Santé, the largest hospital in suburban Laval, Quebec, staff took the unusual step of issuing a press release early in the month. The sick were asked to delay any visit to the hospital.
- In Montreal, nurses at Sacré-Coeur staged a wildcat strike to protest the overcrowding, a problem experienced by every hospital in the city. For instance, at Maisonneuve-Rosemont — a hospital that had drawn national attention the year before because an elderly patient had died while waiting to be seen in its overcrowded emergency room — 79 patients jammed into a room designed to accommodate only 34.

- In Nelson, British Columbia, a 74-year-old ER patient was placed in a hospital storage area. No other room could be found for him at a time when patients were routinely placed in hallways and linen closets. And, in Victoria, facilities were running at 110% capacity — since the summer before.

The above incidents all occurred during a two-week period that was by no means unusual. It's not difficult to find newspaper articles throughout 1999 about physician shortages, long waiting times for treatments, and a lack of high-tech equipment. It doesn't matter which daily newspaper you pick. The problems in Halifax are similar to those in Montreal, Saskatoon, and Vancouver.

Of course, you needn't open a newspaper if you want to hear about the problems with the health care system. Friends and family can relate their own stories.

When such stories come to light, they are almost always underplayed by the so-called experts. A health care consultant told a CBC Newsworld panel that Canadians are far too negative. On the topic of the missed lung transplant, he observed that it's a "miracle" doctors can perform lung transplants at all. "Two out of three [lung transplants in a day] isn't bad," he noted, based on the fact that the Toronto Hospital had performed two lung transplants the morning Smith was scheduled to have his surgery.

Such views are common. Even those who openly criticize the health care system — opposition politicians, union spokespeople, physicians — typically have grievances with the way a provincial government manages the system but not with the basic organization of the system. When medicare is discussed, two opinions are usually expressed. The magicians believe that, with just the right combination of government regulations, medicare will magically work. The spendthrifts argue that more government money would solve every problem — from the attitude of the grumpiest hospital orderly to the lengthiest waiting list for radiation therapy.

Magicians and spendthrifts dominate the health care debate in Canada. And, on the surface, they seem to have little in common. That they attack each other with great contempt in public debates no doubt fosters this view. John Ralston Saul, a writer, explained at the Canadian Medical Association conference The Future of Health Care that "anyone who doesn't think that putting billions of dollars back into the health care system is a good idea is either crazy or in the business of caskets."

Both magicians and spendthrifts, however, believe in a government-run health care system. And, while they don't agree on the best way to reform medicare, they basically agree that government action, whether more spending or better management, will provide a solution.

Provincial governments have been busy implementing the ideas from these two camps. Health care has never been managed more than it is today. For all the talk of "using money better" and "coordinating and integrating," provincial governments have spent the past two decades feverishly implementing one management idea after another: regional health boards, bed closures, and now community care.

Despite the widespread view that health care spending has declined in recent years, it hasn't. In 1990, in the easy deficit-spending days, total health care expenditures amounted to $61 billion. In 1998, after federal Minister of Finance Paul "the Axe" Martin supposedly chopped down the health care budget, more than $80 billion was spent, an increase of about 33% (roughly 20%, factoring in inflation).

Yet medicare is worse than it has ever been. What's going on?

Code Blue attempts to answer this question. On the great debate of our time — more money or better management — this book rejects both ideas. Magicians and spendthrifts are persuasive and well spoken, but the ideas they champion are about as useful as rearranging the deck chairs on the *Titanic*. This book challenges many of the widely accepted "truths" about medicare, including the most important one: medicare is fundamentally sound and is merely in a time of transition.

Chapter 1 details the state of the health care system. Although many Canadians are familiar with polls suggesting widespread public concern (and with the anecdotal evidence behind this concern), the first chapter looks at specific indicators: studies on waiting times for treatments, statistics on high-tech equipment, and physician migration. From the American practice of a frustrated Canadian surgeon to the struggle over Vancouver Island's MRI scanner, the chapter gauges the real state of medicare — and soundly rejects the "don't worry, be happy" attitude of so many health care experts.

Chapter 2 follows the political debate over medicare, offering a careful critique of Reform and Liberal positions. The chapter takes a serious look at the cherished Canada Health Act, promises of pharmacare, and the bidding war over increasing health care funding. It also notes that, while both the government and the opposition are eager to attack one another, their public pronouncements are generally hollow and eerily similar.

Because so much of the health care discussion in Canada focuses on the American system, chapter 3 takes a careful look across the border. It explodes commonly held beliefs: that U.S. health care is free market, that government noninvolvement has resulted in millions of citizens without insurance, and that high administrative costs are inherently wasteful. It also observes, perhaps surprisingly, that the trend in U.S. health care — away from individual choice and toward bureaucratic management — parallels that in medicare.

Chapter 4 looks at the economic problem at the heart of medicare's woes. With no direct cost to the patient, and the physician billing the government, the basic doctor-patient relationship gets distorted. An expensive system full of perverse incentives is the result. To combat these incentives, governments have worked feverishly to save money — largely by restricting patients' access to the care they want and need.

Demographics has become a hot topic in discussions about public policy (e.g., pensions) but not about health care. Chapter 5 explains why health care analysts need to look at demographics. Indeed, Canada's aging population coupled with the rising costs of medical technology is sure to increase pressures on the health care system. Time, it seems, will make medicare's problems much worse, not better.

Chapter 6 takes the observations of previous chapters and weaves them into a series of principles for a good health care system: quality, cost effectiveness, timeliness, consumer orientation, and efficiency. It then looks at alternative proposals — user fees, more money, two-tiered health care, internal markets — and explains why they fall short. The failings of these ideas, however, contrast with the success of society's ability to address other basic needs, such as food, clothing, and shelter.

Chapter 7 outlines a health care system that doesn't fall short on these principles. It's possible not only to preserve universality and accessibility but also to avoid waiting lists and declining standards. Such a system is built on the simple idea that it should be run not by the government but by the people who use it. This chapter details the concept of medical savings accounts and discusses experiments with them in other countries.

The epilogue describes how such a system might work in the future for three generations of a fictional family.

This book, in short, breaks from the typical discussion of health care, which increasingly resembles a tiger chasing its own tail. It's a book written in plain English, free of complicated technical language. And it's an invitation for those in the health care field, patients, and concerned citizens to do what nearly no politician or expert is willing to do: take an honest look at our health care system.

1

A Troubled System

VOCAL CRITICS of Canada's social programs — writers, political activists, and policy analysts — tend to be young and ideological. Concerned about economic growth and taxes, such critics happily quote economist Milton Friedman and read columnist Mark Steyn.

Perhaps this is what makes Bill McArthur such an unlikely critic of the medicare system. A tall, older gentleman with a deep voice, Dr. McArthur could best be described as a gentle giant, the sort of person everyone wants as a family physician.

Dr. McArthur spent 24 years in the Canadian Forces working as a fighter pilot, a physician, and a research scientist. He then set up a private practice and went on to serve as the first chief coroner of British Columbia. Semiretired, today he handles a small practice of palliative care patients, attempting to alleviate the pain and suffering of the dying. And, for the record, McArthur never quotes Friedman.

His own health care experience in 1997 — he had a brush with prostate cancer — helped to confirm his long-standing belief that medicare is deeply flawed. "The BC government doesn't believe that a PSA test [a simple blood test that can detect prostate cancer] is useful," McArthur explained to me in June 1998, referring to the fact that this test is no longer covered by the provincial health insurance. "I figured, if the government doesn't believe in it, there must be something right with the test." After weeks of feeling ill, he underwent the test. It came back positive. McArthur was sick with prostate cancer. "That test probably saved my life."

But if his own health care experience has helped to confirm his views, years of practice have formed them. "In the past," McArthur dryly noted, "we did the best we *could* for patients. Today we do the best we are *allowed* to do under the circumstances."

In particular, waiting lists distress the doctor. He gave as an example the experience of a former patient: "She was in her sixties, independent living. She was active and an excellent gardener. She had terrible back pain. It seemed like a classic presentation of spinal stenosis [a disease in which the spine degenerates and pinches the nerves], so we ordered a CT scan." The diagnostic test, however, was difficult to get. "She was expected to wait three months. The pain was terrible. She would wake up screaming at night. You just can't control that sort of pain with morphine, you know."

McArthur used his connections to speed up the process for this patient. After many phone calls, he arranged that she could get the scan in a month. When the diagnosis was confirmed, he referred her to a surgeon. "The neurosurgeon wanted her to wait 15 months before surgery." Unsatisfied, McArthur started calling around. Finally, he found a young neurosurgeon in another community who was willing to perform the operation — in one month. "The system would have left her in pain for years," McArthur noted with a trace of anger. "Years."

It's the experiences of people like McArthur and his patients that have caused Canadians to realize that the medicare system is not without problems. In a 1999 Angus Reid poll (see Greenspon, "Health Care"), only 24% of Canadians rated the system as "excellent" or "very good." Four years earlier, 52% of Canadians gave the system top marks. In 1991, a full 61% rated the system highly. More and more citizens conclude that the best days of medicare are in the past. A majority of Canadians, according to Angus Reid, believe that the system is going to decline in the coming years.

In a 1998 Pollara survey involving over 3,000 people, 96% agreed that "substantial repairs, if not a complete rebuilding, are necessary to maintain the [health care] system's quality" (Kennedy and Dube). A COMPAS survey in early 1999 found that 79% of respondents view health care services as having declined in the last few years, with 46% judging they had become "much worse" (Gillis).

With such numbers, it's not surprising that health care is quickly emerging as the biggest issue of the day, concerning the polity as much as deficit reduction in the 1980s and early 1990s did. In poll after poll from Angus Reid, it's named as the primary concern of Canadians — ahead of poverty, taxes, and the economy combined (Angus Reid Group).

What lies behind this developing crisis in confidence? Is there really cause for concern?

1.1 Stories of Deficiencies

Part of the reason for the pessimism — or, perhaps, the realism — is that Canadians are increasingly hearing about the system's shortcomings. Newspapers and TV news shows frequently report the problems people encounter with waiting lists and limited equipment. Consider, for example, the following stories that detail in graphic terms the suffering of Canadians. The cases are from major newspapers and magazines such as the *Ottawa Citizen*, the *Globe and Mail*, and *Health Affairs*.

CASE 1

Ladora Schwab, British Columbia

After Ladora Schwab of the small Vancouver Island community of Cedar suffered a heart attack last September [1997], doctors told her the muscle in the heart wall and her aortic valve were both damaged, and her mitral valve was also leaking. Nevertheless, Schwab, then 63, was given a pacemaker and sent home to take her place in line for further testing. . . .

Schwab died of internal hemorrhaging on March 4 [1998], the day after her family celebrated her 64th birthday. She was scheduled to travel to Victoria on March 17 for an angiogram, a pre-surgery test that measures blockages. A combination of heart attack and multiple blood transfusions had left her swollen with excess fluid and struggling to breathe. "It was a terrible thing to have to watch her go like that," says her husband, Ralph. "She couldn't do anything for at least three months." Schwab's internist, Dr. Neils Schwarts, told Mr. Schwab that he could not say if an operation would have saved the life of his wife. "But," says Mr. Schwab, "he did say the weeks of waiting increased the risk of dying." (Parker 10)

CASE 2

Twila Harris, Ontario

Twila Harris has spent the last four months in waiting. "I feel like a convict sitting on death row who was reprieved for a few moments," says the mother of three and grandmother of two. . . . Mrs. Harris has cancer of the colon, a heart condition, and diabetes. If the cancer moves to her lymph nodes, she has been told, there will be nothing doctors can do.

She needs surgery to remove a tumour in her colon. She needs a bed in the intensive-care unit. She needs the doctors to stop cancelling her operation.

Mrs. Harris, 49, was diagnosed with cancer in November and told she needed the operation. . . . Her first operation was scheduled for February 16. [But] her surgery was pushed back to Monday [March 1] at 8 a.m. But with the gurney at the operation room door, she got more bad news. Her surgery was again stopped. . . . With the surgery pushed back to Tuesday, she was let down one more time. Still no room in the ICU. (Trifunov A1)

CASE 3
Donald Lyons, Ontario

Several years after having a hip replacement at St. Michael's Hospital in Toronto, Donald Lyons, a mutual-fund investment manager, was living in unrelenting pain. With one leg 7.5 cm shorter than the other, increasing back problems, and "a terrible limp," Lyons was incredulous when told by his orthopedic surgeon's staff that he would have to wait 18 months for surgery. "You've gotta be kidding," he retorted. But they weren't.

"They just told me to tough it out."

Lyons wouldn't do that. In January 1996, he saw a University of Virginia Medical Center advertisement in *The Globe and Mail*. It promised high-quality hip- and knee-replacement surgery at a reasonable price.

Lyons checked the center's credentials, liked what he heard and decided that forgoing the agony of an 18-month visit was well worth $15,000 (US), the center's all-inclusive price. He immediately went to Charlottesville, met the same day with an orthopedic surgeon and underwent surgery the following morning. Nine days later he was home.

Today, Lyons has nothing but praise and gratitude for the way he was treated. . . . He has one comment about treatment delays in Canada: "Pathetic!" (Korcok, "Excess Demand" 767)

CASE 4
Michael Walker, British Columbia

My incredulity is heightened by recent personal experiences. My friend Stanley Roberts, past president of the Canadian Chamber of Commerce, died just after Christmas a year ago because he waited ten days on a waiting list at Vancouver General Hospital for a computed tomography (CT) scan to determine if the "thing" in his head was a tumour or an abscess. The abscess was found upon autopsy, but what killed him was the wait, since abscesses can usually be cured with antibiotics.

Six weeks ago, I was found to have a large kidney stone lodged in my ureter [a part of the urinary tract that carries urine from the kidney to the bladder]. My extensive travel schedule and the risks associated with a further blockage of the kidney led my urologist to recommend immediate removal. This would be possible with a one-week wait if he used the old technique of direct removal using a "basket" via the penis. The painless process of lithotripsy (Canada has one lipotripter per six million population) would have involved a wait of three weeks — a course not open to me. So, I had the direct removal with the attendant pain and several days of discomfort. The differential discomfort also does not figure in provincial budgets. (Michael Walker, letter 233)

CASE 5

Senator Pat Carney, British Columbia

The waiting period for my scheduled date with the orthopedic surgeon for a minor knee operation is one year less . . . four days. Thank God, it isn't a joint replacement; that would probably take two years.

While the political parties argue about the medicare system, the reality is that we don't have access to one. . . . Instead, we play the waiting game.

I tore the cartilage in my knee after a stupid sailing accident last September [1996]. When, after months of therapy, my physiotherapist referred me for further medical treatment, I called my long-time rheumatologist and was given an appointment in two months time; a new patient would wait four months. "It's easier to see you for lunch," I told him.

It took three weeks to find a surgeon willing to see me at all, given the waiting lists. Then I waited weeks for the actual appointment and queue number.

It is not just me. At a shopping mall, I ran into a person with rheumatoid arthritis. He looked like the Tin Man. His head was neckbraced off his shoulders, and his arms stuck out on each side in casts. Arthritic nodes were threatening to damage his spinal cord. He was excited. He was scheduled to see a neurosurgeon after only a three-month wait!

Another friend's father died in hospital waiting for surgery. After he was declared brain-dead, he qualified as an emergency.

"Don't blame me," said the orthopedic surgeon when I finally met him. "The system only allows me to operate six hours a week. Last year it was 18 hours. . . ."

"And he is a good surgeon," said a friend's gynecologist, whose waiting list is three or four months.

The surgeon said that if I were a Japanese tourist or an American visitor, he might be able to help me. But since I was a Canadian taxpayer, he couldn't. Unless I claimed special or emergency circumstances.

"Why didn't you queue-jump?" he asked. "I don't know how," I answered frankly. He named some professionals who did. They included provincial politicians, labour leaders, university presidents. No names, of course. "How do you think hockey stars get immediate medical attention?" (Carney)

CASE 6

Dr. Steven Levinson, Ontario

"There was a time when I felt that any patient going to hospital would get consistently good care in Canada, but now I feel you have only a 70 or 80 percent chance of getting it," said Dr. Steven Levinson, a Toronto general practitioner, who supports the system but worries about how it has been managed.

Dr. Levinson said his eyes were opened when he had bypass surgery three years ago and found he was getting the wrong medication. When he needed an electrocardiogram, he was forced to wait because one of the only two machines in the hospital was broken. "And when I was in intensive care my feet stuck to the floor it was so dirty," he said. (DePalma)

CASE 7

Harold Yule, Alberta

Calgarian Harold Yule said he went public with his case in a bid to give the province "a wake-up call," but he doubts anyone heard it.

The 52-year-old heavy-equipment operator was turned away from the Bow Valley Centre emergency department last February and advised to go home since the Peter Lougheed Hospital emergency ward was also jammed.

He spent the night in agony at home suffering from a crushed vertebra, broken right heel, shattered left ankle, and broken shin bone before returning to the emergency room by ambulance the next day. Even then, it took six hours before he was admitted. (Henton)

CASE 8

Dr. Bruno L'Heureux, Quebec

[Canadian Medical] Association president Bruno L'Heureux concluded his term in office by recalling advice his mother gave him before she died last year.

"I pity you when your turn comes to be a patient," he recalled her saying. "I hope your beliefs will drive you to improve a dreadful system, one in which we feel treated like children, diminished, and ridiculed." (Dueckert)

CASE 9

Jean Gendron, Manitoba

Jean Gendron has been losing sleep over lengthy waiting lists for medical care for more than two years. Since March, 1996, Gendron has been waiting to see a specialist who can confirm her doctor's diagnosis of sleep apnea — a potentially fatal condition where people stop breathing while they sleep. Without a diagnosis, she cannot get treatment.

After suffering through sleepless nights and days where she cannot go to a movie or drive long distances for fear of falling asleep, Gendron has turned to Ontario for help. She decided to travel to a clinic in Thunder Bay where it took her only a few weeks to get an appointment. . . . "I have to pay my own way and miss three days of work, but it will be worth it."

After two years on a waiting list in Manitoba, Gendron said she still has no idea when she would have got to see a specialist. Her case is not seen as a priority because there is no immediate threat to life. "I'm told they are just getting through the non-priority people from 1995." (Nairne, "Sleep Patient")

Such awful accounts join a growing list of news stories that question the quality and cost of the health care system that Canadians have assumed is simply "the best in the world." Consider the headlines below.

- "Canada's Cancer System Slips to Second Best: As Patients Demand Better Care, Many Top Doctors Warn that the Erosion Must Stop." *Globe and Mail* 25 July 1998.
- "More Medical Specialists Leaving: The Worsening Exodus Means that Patients Are Having to Wait Longer for Some Services, a Physicians' Federation Says." *Gazette* [Montreal] 16 June 1998.
- "Victims of Medicare." *BC Report* 8 June 1998.

- "Crisis Creates Suicide Surge: Mentally Ill Can't Get the Help They Need, Society Official Says." *Winnipeg Free Press* 15 April 1998.
- "Health Care Stressed across Country." *Edmonton Sun* 7 March 1998.
- "Long Wait for Emergency Care: Health Ministry in the Hotseat." *Toronto Sun* 19 February 1998.
- "Growing Waiting List for Heart Surgery a Concern." *Medical Post* 6 January 1998.
- "Three Die While on Heart Waiting List." *Calgary Herald* 25 February 1997.
- "State Health Care Withers." *Winnipeg Free Press* 5 February 1997.
- "Radical Surgery: Canadian Health Care May Be among the Best but Medicare, Barely 30 Years Old, Is Enfeebled by Nationwide 'Reforms' Driven by Bottom-Line Dollar Politics." *Maclean's* 2 December 1996.
- "Can Medicare Be 'Saved'?" *Toronto Star* 1 December 1996.
- "Health System in Crisis: Soaring Costs Put Stress on Nation's Medicare System." *Halifax Chronicle-Herald* 10 October 1996.
- "Medicare: Canadians Have a Reason to Worry about It." *Vancouver Sun* 14 October 1995.
- "Condition Critical as Health System Nears 30." *Toronto Star* 23 September 1995.
- "Canada's Medicare on the Sick-List." *Economist* 23 and 29 September 1995.

Such headlines are troubling. Equally troubling is the fact that news reports suggesting problems with the medicare system are neither recent nor fleeting. Indeed, looking back to the end of the last decade, we find the following.

- "Health System Ill in Quebec, Says Founder." *Ottawa Citizen* 25 January 1990.
- "Bed Closings Blasted: 91 Left on Backlog for Urgent Surgery." *Winnipeg Free Press* 5 July 1989.
- "Ontario's Health Care Is in Critical Condition." *London Free Press* 27 May 1989.
- "Need Surgery, Medical Tests? Go to the End of the Line." *Globe and Mail* 28 May 1988.

*   *   *

These stories point to a health care system plagued by serious problems. Is medicare really in such bad shape? Or are such accounts isolated and rare?

Politicians and health care experts have reviewed the evidence and seem to be satisfied. Politicians of every political stripe have little hesitation in declaring medicare the "best health care system in the world." They are not alone in this view. Indeed, in 1997 the National Forum on Health released its final report after two years of study, at an expense of $10 million. The conclusion: "We believe that the health care system is fundamentally sound" (iv). Forum chair Dr. Tom Noseworthy went so far as to publicly scold the system's critics: "Shame on you for saying there's a crisis!"

When the topic of waiting lists comes up, many of the experts are particularly annoyed. In a *Toronto Star* article, Professors Bob Evans, one of the country's most prominent health economists, and Noralou Roos, chair of a major health care research centre, argue that "Claims of excessive waiting lists are the 'political theatre' of publicly funded health care everywhere in the world" (A11). At the 1998 annual conference of McMaster University's Centre for Health Economics and Policy Analysis, epidemiologist Dr. Charles Wright stated that "the waiting list problem is greatly exaggerated and distorted" (qtd. in Borsellino 29). And a study of waiting times for surgery in Manitoba declares that "Long waits for treatment are frequently viewed as a failure of the health care system. But it is an area where there is far more rhetoric than reality" (De Coster et al. 11). They explore the source of this rhetoric: "Perhaps Canadians' perception of the unduly long waits for surgery are influenced by the rhetoric from south of the border. American critics of a publicly-funded health care system are quick to point out the long waits in Canada and label it as rationing" (11).

In their latest book on the Canadian health care system, *Universal Health Care: What the United States Can Learn from the Canadian Experience*, Carleton University professors Pat Armstrong and Hugh Armstrong support this view: "Canadians do not wait for care that is required immediately" (126). There may be waiting lists for some minor procedures but certainly not for urgent surgeries, they maintain. But why, then, do Canadians believe that waiting lists are a problem? The Armstrongs find an answer that combines American bashing with class envy: "The rich cannot buy their way to the front of the line in the Canadian health care system. A few of them, and some U.S. critics, have as a result taken to complaining about the delays before certain procedures are carried out" (126).

Michael Decter, chair of the Canadian Institute for Health Information, writes in his book *Healing Medicare: Managing Health System Change the Canadian Way* that "We have waiting lists for some procedures as a means of better organizing our system." He even suggests that patients prefer this system since they "often wish to have surgery scheduled in the future" (209).

Finally, in *Strong Medicine: How to Save Canada's Health Care System*, Dr. Michael Rachlis and Carol Kushner dismiss the waiting list problem. They even suggest, in true conspiracy fashion, that where waiting lists do develop for heart surgery the cause has little to do with the health care system and much to do with greedy physicians: doctors, they explain, deliberately keep patients waiting for treatment in order to blackmail governments into increasing health care funding.

Far from being the exception, such comments on waiting lists and times are often repeated by policy analysts, health economists, and politicians. The so-called experts are quick to dismiss the entire problem of waiting for treatment, arguing either that waiting lists do not exist or that, if they do, the waits are insignificant and local in nature.

It just doesn't add up. Are Canadians being misled by an overzealous — or, perhaps, sensationalistic — press corps?

Despite the vigour with which experts and politicians defend the present system, there is a significant body of anecdotal evidence that medicare is seriously troubled. Perhaps more importantly, the limited statistical and demographic information available on medicare and Canada's population indicates that many problems exist in the system. Despite adamant assurances from the experts, Canadians should recognize that the system is in bad shape. Patients are suffering.

But we need to clarify the point. Sometimes people — including members of the media — confuse bad care with bad medicare. When patients are poorly treated, they may be tempted to blame the system. Yet a doctor with a poor bedside manner doesn't necessarily reflect on the success or failure of medicare. Nor does a misdiagnosis in the emergency room by an incompetent physician. Nor does the carelessness of a sloppy orderly.

A meaningful analysis of the medicare system will recognize that bad doctoring is not bad medicare. That bad nursing is not bad medicare. Even the best-organized health care system will have its share of incompetent physicians, nurses, orderlies, and technicians. But, bearing this in mind, does the medicare system make it easier or harder for competent and conscientious staff to do the best job they can? It is increasingly clear that medicare as it is currently organized undermines the quality of care patients receive.

It's not surprising to learn, then, that the people who have the most intimate knowledge of the system — the doctors — are the most pessimistic about the quality of care being provided. Responding to the Canadian Medical Association's 1998 Physician Resource Questionnaire, doctors were troubled by access to care. Only 27% of physicians rated as excellent, very good, or good their access to advanced diagnostic equipment such as MRI scanners. Also in other areas, few physicians were willing to give the system top marks for access: long-term institutional care (30%), psychosocial support services (45%), and acute institutional care for elective procedures (45%). Even in cases involving urgent care, physicians didn't give medicare a ringing endorsement: only 63% rated "acute institutional care on an urgent basis" as between excellent and good (CMA 12).

Moving beyond polls, three areas are particularly troublesome: the waiting lists, the exodus of physicians, and the technology gap. The following sections will explore these areas.

1.2 Waiting for Care

Canadians are often forced to wait a long time before receiving treatment. Occasionally, the waiting can have dire consequences. Consider the following horror stories, cited by Joseph Weber. Jeyaraanie Kaneshakumar, in her eighth month of pregnancy, died of a brain hemorrhage. Suspecting a neurological problem, doctors had wanted to admit her but couldn't find a neurosurgical facility to take her. She was 35. Jean-François Giguère-Bélisle died in 1997 after his ruptured appendix went undiagnosed in two clinics and an emergency room. He was only 10 years old. Frances Lever, 49, died after her stomach pains turned out to be cancer. Treatment was delayed for weeks because of cancelled appointments and a misdiagnosis.

These are rare examples, but there is significant anecdotal evidence that waiting lists exist for even the most common tests and treatments. In November 1996, *Maclean's* printed a sharp piece by John DeMont. After quoting a Reform Party staffer who praised the medicare system, DeMont writes:

> He might sound different if he had a child with a chronic ear infection
> who had to wait 11 months for an appointment to have a myrighotomy (an

alleviating surgical procedure in which a tube is inserted through the tympanic membrane). Or if he had to wait seven months — the norm in Ottawa at the moment — for a hip replacement, six months for non-urgent cardiac surgery, four weeks for an appointment with a hospital psychiatrist, or two months for a neurologist. (63–64)

During the 1996 doctors' strike in Ontario, physicians often complained about the lengthy waiting lists. Dr. Gerry Rowland, then president of the Ontario Medical Association, suggested that the strike was "a rescue mission" because the system was in real trouble. The fact that people are forced to wait up to two years for hip-replacement surgery was used as an example ("OMA").

My own views on waiting lists have been darkly coloured by the experiences of a few family friends: a young Winnipeg woman with severe abdominal pain was expected to wait six months for the pain-alleviating gall bladder surgery; a community college teacher from southern Ontario suffered heart trouble and was forced to take a year off work while he waited for bypass surgery; an older woman with severe sleeping problems was put on a two-year waiting list to see a respiratory specialist.

But such anecdotal evidence doesn't reveal the extent of the problem. To judge the gravity of the waiting list situation, we need more information. How many people are on waiting lists? How long do they typically wait? Does waiting cause them physical discomfort or limit them in some way? Are the waiting lists getting shorter or longer? What are the consequences of this waiting period for the patient and for our society?

Waiting Your Turn

"Official" data on waiting lists are not comprehensive. Unlike in the United Kingdom, where local governments carefully track the waiting periods, most provinces do not keep such information. There are, however, a few nongovernment studies. Of them, the Fraser Institute publishes the most comprehensive work: *Waiting Your Turn: Hospital Waiting Lists in Canada*, by Cynthia Ramsay and Michael Walker.

In this annual study, physicians of 12 medical specialties are surveyed: plastic surgery, gynecology, ophthalmology, otolaryngology, general surgery, neurosurgery, orthopedic surgery, cardiovascular surgery, urology, internal medicine, radiation oncology, and medical oncology. Specialists in these areas are asked a series of questions that attempt to determine the length of two different types of waiting: the wait between a referral from a family physician to the specialist, and the wait from the specialist to the necessary diagnostic test or surgery. Specialists are also asked what they consider to be a "reasonable number of weeks to wait" before the necessary treatment is started.

Many dismiss this study because it is done by a group perceived to be "right-wing." When asked about studies of waiting lists, for example, a former CMA president told me that "The Fraser Institute does something, but it is the Fraser Institute."

But the assumption that *Waiting Your Turn* is tainted by bias is inaccurate. Listening to critics of the study, we might think that the data are based on a sampling of carefully selected patients and physicians united by their displeasure with medicare. This simply isn't the case. The study is based on information gathered from Canada's medical specialists. There is no prescreening. *Waiting Your Turn* reflects the answers given by these physicians to uniform and carefully worded questions.

The analysis that accompanies the data provides an unbiased assessment of the survey results: observations about the findings, description of methodology, and so on. In the entire 60-page publication, only one section (one page in length) provides an argument that could be perceived as controversial. Whether the economic argument that non-price rationing is inferior to price rationing reflects an ideological bias or a reasoned conclusion based on sound economic analysis is debatable. In any case, the section on price rationing in no way influences the value of the results or undermines the credibility of the data. *Waiting Your Turn* deserves serious consideration.

The survey itself was originally developed in 1990 with the help of the BC Medical Association as a means of measuring waiting lists in British Columbia. Based on input from a variety of sources, including the Canadian Hospital Association (now the Canadian Healthcare Association), participating physicians, and others, the survey's scope and analysis have been expanded. Today the survey covers all 10 provinces and boasts a response rate of about a quarter of all Canadian specialists.

The results indicate, for example, that the total waiting time for a hernia patient in British Columbia is about nine weeks. Consider the following scenario. A man living in Vancouver goes to his family physician complaining that, after moving his belongings into a new apartment, he has a sharp pain in his lower abdomen. The pain has persisted for a few days and bothers him all the time, even though he is taking aspirin. The physician asks a variety of questions, inspects the man's abdomen, and concludes that the patient has a hernia. He then refers the man to a general surgeon. According to the survey, the patient has to wait a couple of weeks before he sees the surgeon. The surgeon then looks him over, asks him some more detailed questions, and concludes that, yes, he does have a hernia that requires minor surgery. If the patient agrees to go ahead with the operation, thereby ending his ailment and the physical discomfort associated with it, he will have to wait seven more weeks. In other words, the total waiting period from initial pain to surgical treatment is over two months.

It may seem surprising that even a minor, uncomplicated operation such as a hernia repair is subject to a long wait. But this is the tip of the iceberg — the Fraser Institute study suggests that waiting times plague every aspect of health care, from minor procedures to urgent surgeries. Following is a summary of the major findings.

1. In 1997, there were over 187,000 Canadians waiting for surgical procedures. The study notes that, according to a Statistics Canada paper, 45% of patients waiting for treatment describe themselves as being "in pain."[1] While treatment may not necessarily alleviate this pain, the implication is clear — waiting prolongs physical suffering for many patients.

2. There were 8.5% more patients on waiting lists in 1997 than in the previous year. Those patients also tended to wait longer: 11.9 weeks from general practitioner referral, up from 9.3 weeks in 1993.

3. Waiting times for treatment affected patients in every medical specialty. Ophthalmologic (eye) surgery, orthopedic (bone and joint) surgery, elective cardiac (heart) surgery, and neurosurgery (brain, spine, and nerve) patients waited the longest: 24.6, 20.7, 18.2, and 16.5 weeks respectively.

4. Responding specialists thought that patients were forced to wait too long for treatment in each specialty.

5. Waiting times differed greatly between the provinces. Saskatchewan had the longest period between a visit to the general practitioner and the start of treatment (17.1 weeks), Ontario the shortest (10.2 weeks).

6. Compared with 1967, when a similar survey was done by the British Columbia Hospital Insurance Service, the median waiting time in British Columbia has increased from five weeks to nine weeks in 1995.

7. There is a serious problem with waiting times for cardiovascular surgery.[2] Five of the nine provinces where these operations are performed have waiting times for "emergent" surgeries that fall outside the safe period, as

defined by an Ontario panel of cardiovascular surgeons in 1991.[3] For "urgent" cardiac surgery, British Columbia falls outside the range. And for "elective" cardiac surgery, New Brunswick and Newfoundland are beyond the recommended period of six months.

Such findings are damning. Can it be that over 150,000 citizens are waiting for treatment, many of them in physical pain? These statements stand in strong contrast to the analysis made by vocal (and established) proponents of medicare. The final report of the National Forum on Health, for example, mentions waiting lists only in passing, not even suggesting they are a problem; the problem is that "people are told by the media that waiting lists are getting longer" (9).

A huge gap exists between what the experts think about the waiting list issue — and, by extension, the system as a whole — and what the Fraser Institute suggests with its study. It's not surprising, then, that the experts are harsh in their criticism of the study.

Critics suggest that the findings are flawed because physicians are not a reliable source of information — specialists do not submit seriously considered answers, or, worse, they deliberately and cynically inflate their numbers in an attempt to justify increased health care funding. A government-sponsored report by Health Canada even suggests that "waiting lists are inflated by 20 percent to 30 percent (and often more) by the presence of those who have died, receiving the procedure, no longer wish to have the procedure or do not know they are scheduled" (McDonald et al. 13).

The charge has some merit. It's conceivable that some physicians would skew their data. But there is as much reason for a doctor to inflate data — a dishonest (and round-about) attempt to influence health care funding — as there is to misreport data in the other direction — an attempt to suggest that the physician's patients are well taken care of or that the practice is particularly efficient.

In fact, there really isn't much evidence to support the claim that physicians deliberately and grossly misrepresent the situation. The much-quoted Health Canada statistic — that 20% to 30% of waiting lists is padding — is based on an international literature review. The authors of the study could not offer any proof that such practices exist in Canada.

Rather than debating the reasons for physician fudging, it makes more sense to compare the data collected by the Fraser Institute with a smaller and more focused analysis of the waiting list issue. Doing so isn't easy, though; for the most part, provincial governments keep relatively little information on waiting times for treatment. Still, in limited areas, official data are available. And, if anything, *Waiting Your Turn* can be faulted for underestimating the duration of waiting. Consider the Fraser Institute study in relation to government data in the following three jurisdictions.

1. *Newfoundland and Labrador.* The Department of Health and Community Services collected average waits and the number of patients in various specialties. For the most part, the Fraser Institute's survey findings fall within the range provided by the department, though *Waiting Your Turn* tends to estimate waiting times toward the lower part of the official data. For orthopedic surgery, for example, the Fraser Institute estimated a wait of 4.6 weeks, and the Department of Health and Community Services gave a range of from six to 24 weeks.

2. *Alberta.* The Ministry of Health kept information on joint-replacement surgery and cardiovascular surgery. The data suggested that 800 patients were waiting for joint surgery. The Fraser Institute survey reported only 638 patients.

3. *Quebec.* Data from the Montreal Regional Health Board showed 377 patients waiting for heart surgery in March 1997. The Fraser Institute study estimated 359.

In areas where available data cannot be directly compared with the Fraser Institute's work, the news isn't good. The British Columbia Cancer Agency (BCCA), for example, suggests that patients should wait a maximum of two weeks from referral to specialist and then a maximum of two weeks from specialist to treatment. This is the agreed-upon standard for radiation oncology. BCCA data from April 1998 suggest that the care of a majority of patients fails to meet the standard. At the Vancouver centre, only 47% of patients received radiation therapy within the two-week time frame. On Vancouver Island, 49% of patients fell within the proper time period. The Fraser Valley centre had better results: 91% of patients were treated in a timely manner.

Critics have also questioned how physicians interpret waiting times. The Fraser Institute asks specialists not only how long their patients wait but also how long they think their patients should wait. Certainly, critics have argued, physician subjectivity influences the result.

Again, though, the available evidence doesn't support the criticism. Indeed, conversations with Canadian physicians reveal the surprising extent to which waiting times have become an accepted and acceptable part of the system. Doctors don't excessively fret about patients waiting months for CT scans or MRIs. Dr. W.J. Mackillop and his group of analysts at the Radiation Oncology Research Unit at Queen's University observed physicians' desensitization when comparing waiting times for radiation treatment in Canada and the United States. Radiotherapy is a popular treatment for several types of carcinomas (cancers). Mackillop and his colleagues asked the heads of radiation oncology at all cancer centres listed by the International Union Against Cancer in Canada and the United States about the medically acceptable waiting time for radiotherapy from referral to the start of treatment (Mackillop, Zhou, and Quirt). For five of the six scenarios, Canadian specialists tolerated longer waits. In the case of bone metastases, for example, Canadian department heads — compared with their American counterparts — were willing to tolerate waiting times twice as long. Only in the emergency of spinal cord compression did the doctors from the two countries agree on what is acceptable. Apparently, Canadian doctors have become tolerant of long waiting times.

The Fraser Institute study isn't flawless. As with any study that relies on survey data, small sample sizes throw off the results. It's not surprising, then, that data comparisons with Prince Edward Island's Health and Community Services Agency, for instance, weren't at all accurate.

Waiting Your Turn shouldn't be accepted as absolute truth. It is, after all, just a crude measurement of the waiting problem in Canada. The finding that over 187,000 Canadians are waiting for some type of medical service is a rough estimate. Still, the Fraser Institute study is useful. First, the findings suggest that practically any specialty care requires a period of waiting. Second, the specialists providing the care believe that these waiting periods are far too long and may have a detrimental impact on the health of the patient. And third, despite years of health care reforms, waiting lists have not gone away — in fact, the problem seems to be worsening.

Other Studies

Other studies demonstrate that waiting lists are increasingly prevalent and problematic. Dr. W.J. Mackillop and his group at the Queen's Radiation Oncology Research Unit, for instance, conducted a study of the waiting times for radiotherapy at seven Ontario cancer centres. The

study, "Waiting for Radiotherapy in Ontario," compiled data from 1982
to 1991 on patients suffering from carcinoma of the larynx, cervix, lung,
and prostate. Additionally, it collected data on the postoperative use of
radiotherapy for breast cancer patients. Following are the findings of
the study.[4]

1. There were significant variations in median waiting times between the
   various cancer centres.
2. Median waiting times for radiotherapy in Ontario grew steadily between
   1982 and 1991. The wait from diagnosis to the start of curative treatment
   for laryngeal cancer, cervical cancer, non-small cell lung cancer, and prostate cancer increased by 178.1%, 105.6%, 158.3%, and 62.9% respectively.
   Waiting times for the start of radiotherapy for postoperative breast cancer
   patients increased by 102.7%.
3. In 1982, the bulk of patients began treatment within the time line recommended by the Committee on Standards of the Canadian Association of
   Radiation Oncologists; by 1991, few patients received care within the prescribed intervals. The authors note that

   > Long delays in starting radiotherapy are clearly not good for our pa-
   > tients. . . . Treatment delays which may exceed the doubling time of
   > some common malignancies decrease the probability of local control,
   > and increase the probability of metastasis outside the treatment field,
   > although the magnitude of these risks remains to be established and
   > will vary depending on the specific clinical situation. (11)
4. The magnitude of the problem is underestimated by the study results. For
   technical reasons, the data from one of the centres were excluded for
   1989–91, meaning that the actual waiting lists are longer than reported. As
   well, the long waiting lists meant that some physicians chose alternative —
   and possibly less successful — treatments for their patients, thereby underestimating the magnitude of the problem.

Mackillop's study can be added to a growing list of studies of and
reports on waiting lists and waiting times. Consider the following.

- A study on heart surgery, published in the *Canadian Medical Association
  Journal*, examined coronary heart bypass grafting, or heart bypass surgery, in
  Newfoundland and Labrador from 1994 to 1995 (Fox, O'Dea, and Parfrey).
  Bypass procedures are commonly performed in people with severe coro-
  nary artery disease. The surgery not only improves the quality of life —
  patients no longer suffer from angina chest pains — but also increases life

expectancy. The study attempted to determine the timeliness of care, and the findings are startling. Of the 31 patients who required "very urgent" surgery, only 7 (23%) got the bypass within the recommended period of 24 hours. Of the 122 patients who required "urgent" surgery, only 30 (24%) went into the operating room within the recommended 72 hours. And, to make matters worse, the waiting list increased by 20% during the study period. As the authors conclude, "Failure to perform them [the surgeries] quickly in urgent cases may contribute to excess illness, unnecessary hospital costs, and patient dissatisfaction" (1142).

- The *Winnipeg Free Press* reported in April 1998 that, according to government documents, 12% of women in Manitoba who are ultimately diagnosed with breast cancer through mammograms wait more than 16 weeks for tests to confirm malignancies. That's eight times longer than the international standard (Paul).

- Programs of psychiatric treatment are similarly limited by lengthy waiting lists. Based on a survey of Canadian psychiatrists, Dr. Blake Woodside and Dr. Elizabeth Lin estimated in a presentation to the American Psychiatric Association that patients typically wait an average of two months for a first appointment (Gadd). In Manitoba, the Society of Depression and Manic Depression complained that some treatment programs had waiting periods of six months. In the spring of 1998, it blamed the long waits for the suicides of two depressed patients who couldn't get the help they needed (Nairne, "Crisis"). In Ontario, cash-strapped regional mental health agencies complain that they must routinely refuse patients. "We quite often give them bus tickets to go to Toronto because we don't know where else they could go," said Nancy Roxborough, the executive director of Colborne Community Services (qtd. in Wallace).

- A study that followed 739 breast cancer patients at the three McGill University hospitals between January 1992 and December 1993 found that waiting times were unacceptably high. The study looked at the waiting time for radiation therapy after surgery in early breast cancer. Its conclusion: more than half of the patients waited longer than the recommended time intervals (Benk et al. 115).

- A study presented to the American Association of Orthopedic Surgeons compared patients undergoing total hip- and total knee-replacement surgery at two hospitals: one in Montreal, the other in Boston. Six months after surgery, the Montreal patients fared far worse even though they tended to get more expensive rehabilitation. One reason for the discrepancy was the lengthy waits patients in Canada experienced before they were treated.

Noted the study's author: "It appears surgery may be done too late in the natural history of osteoarthritis at the hospital [Montreal General]" (Wysong).

- In another study by Dr. Mackillop and his colleagues, the heads of radiation oncology at all cancer centres listed by the International Union Against Cancer in Canada and the United States were asked how long patients waited for treatment in six clinical scenarios. There was a significant difference between the ways in which Canadian and American patients were treated. A patient with carcinoma of the larynx waited 29 days for radiation in Canada but just 10 days in the United States. Indeed, for all but emergency treatment, Canadian patients waited far longer than their American counterparts: for carcinoma of the lung, 34 days versus 9 days; for carcinoma of the prostate, 40 days versus 11 days; and for carcinoma of the breast, 43 days versus 10 days. The majority of radiation oncologists in Canada and the United States regarded the delays reported by the Canadian departments as medically unacceptable (Mackillop, Zhou, and Quirt). When Mackillop, a determined advocate of medicare, was called before a U.S. congressional committee and asked what he would do if he had cancer, he replied: "I would go to Buffalo or someplace else in the U.S. to get prompt treatment" (qtd. in Michael Walker, "Canadians").

- Dr. David Bell, an assistant professor of urology at Dalhousie University, and his colleagues presented the preliminary data from a study they are conducting at the 1998 Canadian Urological Association's annual meeting. Bell and his group looked at waiting times for the diagnosis and treatment of patients with gross hematuria (bloody urine), a problem that may indicate cancer. The researchers collected data from two tertiary-care centres in Canada and two similar centres in the United States for a year. Proper diagnosis and follow-up took 20–30 days longer in Canada than in the United States. In Halifax, mean waiting times were 14 days for the referral to the urologist, 19 days for upper tract imaging, 26 days for cystoscopy, 42 days for a CT scan, and 73 days for surgery. "There is no doubt with tumours," observed Bell, "that delay in treatment could affect outcome" (qtd. in Moulton).

- Dr. Fotini Sampalis, a Montreal surgeon, presented to the 1998 annual meeting of the Royal College of Physicians and Surgeons his findings from a survey involving 280 heart surgery patients at three Montreal hospitals. Patients forced to wait 98 days or more, rather than 53 days or fewer, were over three times more likely to have a postsurgery stroke and seven times more likely to have a heart attack. Patients waiting for 98 days or more also experienced reduced physical functioning and vitality, greater job losses, and more complications. "Patients are suffering because of waiting times," observed Sampalis (qtd. in Lem).

- In 1996-97, researchers at the Ontario-based Institute for Clinical Evaluative Sciences (ICES) found that 17% of all Ontario hip-replacement patients and 20% of Ontario knee-replacement patients waited more than 12 months for surgery. Some waited as long as three years. "This is too long," said Dr. J. Ivan Williams, CEO of the ICES and a coauthor of the study (qtd. in Quinn). The 1996 Ontario Expert Panel on Hip and Knee Arthoplasty recommended that all patients, regardless of the levels of pain and disability, shouldn't wait more than 12 months for surgery. Williams noted that currently it isn't known whether waiting a year or two for surgery decreases the chance of an optimal result. The Canadian and Ontario Orthopedic Associations maintain that patients shouldn't have to wait longer than 120 days.

- AAPROACH, a study that looked at 6,000 heart patients from four tertiary-care hospitals in Calgary and Edmonton, found significant problems with the treatment of high-risk patients. Notes the study's author, cardiologist Merril Knudtson: "Heart surgery patients in all centres died more often than predicted. They are treated with medications far too long and go to surgery in a condition that renders their surgical risk higher" (qtd. in Robert Walker, "Alberta"). He estimates that 40 patient deaths could have been avoided in 1995.

- In July 1998, the *Globe and Mail* interviewed administrators from six provincial cancer agencies. The newspaper reminded readers that the Canadian Association of Radiation Oncologists recommends that a cancer patient wait no longer than two weeks to see an oncologist after referral and no longer than two weeks to begin radiation therapy after seeing an oncologist. Although emergency patients were seen in a timely manner, every agency reported a problem with other patients. Those in Nova Scotia typically waited from four to six weeks to begin treatment, some as long as eight weeks. Ontario patients seem to fair the worst: half of all patients wait seven weeks for their first appointment with an oncologist. Two-thirds of patients waited up to eight weeks to begin radiation therapy. Dr. Bernard Cummings, head of Princess Margaret's Department of Radiation Oncology, estimated in a *Toronto Star* interview six months later that only 20% of Ontario patients are seen in the recommended period of four weeks. In comparison, when a survey found that in Britain only 80% of patients were meeting a similar standard, "that was considered a national disgrace" (Daly). Dr. Peter Craighead, director of radiation oncology at Tom Baker Cancer Centre in Calgary, observes: "It's counter intuitive to wait for treatment for cancer. You're taught to screen for cancers and find it early, and then you are told to wait for treatment" (qtd. in Abraham and Fine).

1.3 What Waiting Means

Waiting is an accepted and unavoidable part of daily life. We order a pizza by phone and expect it to be delivered in 45 minutes. We buy a major appliance and know that the delivery truck will not come by for a few days. We order a book through a catalogue and understand that the phrase "four to six weeks" usually means six weeks. Such waiting periods are minor inconveniences. If we had our way, the pizza would be at the door, fresh and piping hot, before we put the phone down. But this is hardly realistic — or, for that matter, important.

Waiting periods for medical diagnosis and treatment are more serious. There are five significant consequences.

1. *Poorer Health*

As suggested by the Canada–US study of joint-replacement surgery, waiting for surgery can have a detrimental effect on health. This isn't surprising — when treatment is delayed, conditions can worsen. Diseases will inflict more damage on the body over time.

Even when a disease is relatively stable, it may negatively impact on other aspects of well-being. An orthopedic surgeon from British Columbia describes as an example a 78-year-old woman requiring a total knee replacement: "Two weeks before the surgery, she was walking down the stairs and her knee jarred from the arthritis. She fell down the stairs and broke her hip."

How often does a delay in treatment result in poorer health? It's difficult to tell, but as waiting lists increase more and more patients are expected to wait longer — often longer than their physicians believe is acceptable. Will an urgent bypass patient really get sicker if his surgery is performed in five days instead of three? Will a breast cancer patient have a poorer prognosis if her radiation therapy begins after eight weeks instead of two? No one is sure, but in these cases treatment is beyond the time periods recommended by the relevant (national) professional body. This doesn't necessarily mean that patients will suffer, but the delays may be detrimental to their health. Given the choice between erring on the side of caution and erring on the side of recklessness, we are increasingly opting for the latter.

And the waiting associated with diagnostic testing is not a positive development. Patients now wait for practically any test, ranging from a lymph node biopsy to a CT scan. Again, such delays aren't necessarily harmful, but every day that a patient waits for a diagnostic test is one more day of waiting to find out what the diagnosis is — and one more day of waiting before treatment can begin. What was the impact on health when, for example, Newfoundland had a shortage of laboratory equipment and "urgent" Pap smears took two months (Goodman and Musgrave 492)? Such waiting periods mean that cancer can go undetected for weeks, possibly months — time for the disease to spread to other organs.

2. Constant Fear

It's difficult for most of us to fully appreciate what life can be like on a waiting list. Blessed with good health, we simply take life for granted. But some aren't so fortunate. For tens of thousands of patients, the wait can mean days, weeks, or even months of agonizing fear.

Will the treatment come too late? Is the cancer spreading? Will my heart give up before I get to the operating room? These questions run through the minds of some patients on waiting lists every hour of every day. No study can quantify their anxiety. No physician or administrator or politician can fully comprehend the terror. For some patients, though, it is a daily reality.

"I wasn't thrilled," explained Miriam Weidman about her ordeal. It's no wonder — for months, she worried about her brain aneurysm. "I learned how to take these things. If that's the way it's got to be, that's the way it's got to be."

At 49, Weidman developed a brain aneurysm as she worked to complete her doctorate in psychology. Before the condition could be treated, the blood vessel burst and caused cerebral hemorrhaging (a stroke). It took many years for her to regain her strength. Years filled with physiotherapy and basic exercises so that she could learn to speak, read, and walk. Then, when she was 71, the original symptoms returned. Fearing the worst, Weidman consulted her doctor. She was referred to a neurosurgeon. It was two months before she could have an MRI to judge the size of the aneurysm. When she finally had the test, the doctor told her the bad news: "the aneurysm was the size of the first one." Still, it took about four more months before she finally had the needed operation. "You have to wait your turn. I realized if this is it, this is it." Then she added, "I was concerned it would burst before I got there."

Thankfully, Weidman was successfully treated. Asked if she was bitter about the experience, she replied firmly: "I don't expect more; the whole thing is dismal."

Even when patients are told that the waiting will not affect their health, the long wait can be a nerve-wracking experience. Consider a woman waiting a full month to get a breast biopsy to determine if the lump is cancerous. Yes, her physician has insisted that, according to the latest epidemiological research, the outcome won't be influenced by such a delay. But does that make the wait any less agonizing?

Many patients must face this fear. Too many.

3. *Suffering and Diminished Quality of Life*

For some patients, a delay in treatment means a delay in the alleviation of pain. Waiting lists, then, are hardly minor inconveniences for these patients — the long wait prolongs suffering.

In 1993, the Institute for Clinical Evaluative Studies at the University of Toronto released a study categorizing the pain endured by patients waiting for hip replacements (Williams and Naylor). The study found that in Ontario 40% of the patients who experienced severe disability and 40% with severe pain were forced to wait more than 13 months for the surgery they needed. Another 40% of those in severe pain waited 7–12 months. Only 14% of the patients in severe pain waited less than four months.

Even when patients aren't in pain, the wait can prolong physical limitations associated with illness. Many patients waiting for a hip replacement have reduced mobility. It can manifest itself in several ways: an end to shopping trips, days of confinement in the apartment, fewer opportunities to visit the grandchildren. The patient's independence and active lifestyle are essentially put on a waiting list. Quality of life diminishes.

This aspect of waiting lists is cruel. Looking for a way out of their predicament, these patients instead find themselves trapped for months, possibly years. This situation is unfair for anyone, but it is particularly unfair for the elderly, for such waits mean that many spend their few remaining days in pain or with physically limiting disabilities. For a 73-year-old woman, a year waiting for a hip replacement may mean that a third of the rest of her life is diminished in quality. One elderly man explained that the long wait had broken his heart. After years of saving for a road trip upon retirement, he instead found himself at the end of a waiting list. "It's not right," he complained.

It's difficult to tell what effect waiting lists have on the overall health of the population. Defenders of medicare are quick to point out that life expectancy is historically at a high. But other statistics provide evidence of a more negative trend. Recent analysis indicates that we are living longer than we were two decades ago, but the number of years that we can expect to live in good health has noticeably declined. According to the Organization for Economic Cooperation and Development, between 1978 and 1991 the number of years a Canadian woman lives in good health (her good-health life expectancy, as defined by the OECD) dropped by 2.3 years. Canadian men also experienced a modest decline of 0.4 years of good health. In contrast, many countries (e.g., France, Switzerland, and the Netherlands) have experienced impressive increases.

The Fraser Institute study argues that there is a link between waiting lists and this trend:

> It has long been known that when rationing emerges in a health care system, the elderly are the most likely to feel the impact. The reason is that in a classic triage system [where priority is given to those who can benefit the most in years], older patients tend to get placed at the end of the queue as they will benefit less from treatment. (Ramsay and Walker 7)

To support this claim, the authors cite articles in the *International Journal of Health Sciences* and the *Medical Post* as well as a presentation made to the Canadian Association on Gerontology.

The findings of a 1995 Ontario study bolster this claim — family physicians, the study found, aren't referring sick and elderly patients as readily as they should for kidney dialysis. "We found substantial evidence of non-referral," says Dr. David Mendelssohn, a nephrologist at the Toronto Hospital. "Some people are not offered a fair choice and are at risk of death" (qtd. in "As Health System Shrinks").

Increasingly, doctors must fight to get their patients the care they need. Faced with lengthy waiting lists for many tests, few hospital beds for admission, and limited operating room time, more and more doctors are finding that patient care involves struggling with administrators and technicians. When patients are particularly old or sick, it's conceivable that doctors are less willing to expend the energy. Perhaps this is why, when the *Globe and Mail* asked Dr. Mark Bernstein, head of the Toronto Hospital's neurosurgery division, to illustrate the aggressiveness of cancer treatment in Canada, he drew a two-centimetre line to illustrate the present effort. He considered a three-centimetre line to be acceptable (Fine).

4. *Financial and Economic Loss*

No studies have been conducted on the financial losses experienced by patients on waiting lists. Such an analysis would be difficult. But there is no question that the long wait for treatment does hit a patient in the wallet.

Cardiologists have long noted that the lengthy wait for heart operations means financial troubles for their patients. After all, the drugs needed to help stabilize the situation can have side effects such as fatigue, dizziness, and general lethargy. Dr. David Gould, head of cardiology in Sault Ste. Marie, noted with concern that patients waiting for surgery "remain sedentary, [and] they sometimes lose their jobs."

Dr. Brian Day, an orthopedic surgeon in Vancouver, believes that a quarter of his patients who wait a year or more require some form of assistance, such as wage-loss benefits or welfare. "They will lose a year's salary when the surgery would be $700," he observed.

Even patients waiting for less dramatic surgeries or basic diagnostic tests have problems. Faced with constant pain or health concerns, they have difficulty maintaining their usual quality of work. Will a report on sales in the third quarter really be the top priority for a business executive who must wait three months to see a neurologist in order to get the numbness in his left arm examined? Can he be expected to pay full attention at his early-morning business meeting after yet another sleepless night spent agonizing about the possibility of a brain tumour? Will he really be able to look after his clients' needs when every night he has nightmares about dying before his children are old enough to take care of themselves?

It's impossible to tell how much money is lost to our economy as a result of the lost employment and productivity. There is, of course, an ironic element to this predicament. Medicare, after all, was introduced so that financial concerns would never have to worry a patient when seeking medical treatment. With a state-run plan, we shouldn't have to think about such things as lost wages and productivity (excluding the unavoidable recovery time), never mind the possibility of losing a job. True, the medicare system means that no one will go bankrupt paying for a life-saving operation, but the waiting lists mean that some people may go bankrupt because of excessive time away from work. And medicare is supposed to ensure that our society will minimize the loss to the economy — with a comprehensive government program, productivity should be maximal. It isn't.

5. Death from Waiting

Many patients who wait for treatment are seriously ill. Some are near death. The waiting list, then, can pose a serious hazard to their lives — if they are forced to wait too long, they may die before receiving the necessary life-saving treatments. Doctors and administrators have attempted to limit the fatalities resulting from the many waiting lists. Using models developed by epidemiologists, they evaluate and then rank patients for surgeries such as heart bypass operations. The sicker the patient, the higher the priority for treatment.

But no model for evaluation is perfect. The severity of a patient's condition can be misjudged. Hence, despite the efforts, some patients have simply fallen through the cracks and died. Others have ranked higher on the waiting lists but, because of the huge backlog for treatment, still waited too long and died. In British Columbia, the case of Philip Georgiou seems to fall into this latter category. His story gathered some local media attention.

> Last October 30 [1997] Philip Georgiou of Kelowna, 61, went to the emergency room of Kelowna General Hospital complaining of discomfort in his chest. An angiogram revealed severe arterial blockages, as well as a floating blood clot. Doctors in Kelowna decided he needed immediate surgery; they wanted to fly him to St. Paul's Hospital in Vancouver.
>
> However, no beds were available and Georgiou was forced to wait until November 5 before going to St. Paul's. "He was scheduled for surgery on November 6," reports his wife Gwen. "But the next day he was bumped by someone more 'urgent.' 'It'll be tomorrow,' they said. Tomorrow stretched into another day, and then another. The whole time my husband was

becoming increasingly nervous and agitated," Mrs. Georgiou recalls. On November 11, she learned by phone that her husband had suffered cardiac arrest and was undergoing emergency surgery. By the time she arrived at the hospital her husband was dead. (Parker 10)

Such incidents rarely come to public attention. In February 1997, a cardiologist in Ontario was so frustrated with the heart surgery situation that he wrote to the provincial minister of health. Dr. David Gould, head of cardiology in Sault Ste. Marie, explained that three northern Ontario patients on a heart bypass waiting list had died within the previous two weeks, and he warned that, with over 250 patients waiting, more deaths could occur ("Three Die").

Occasionally, waiting lists can produce a small crisis in which many people die within a relatively short period of time. The ensuing media attention and the strong public outcry prompt the relevant provincial government to appoint an inquiry or to allocate emergency funds to alleviate the situation. Such was the case, for example, in the late 1980s in Ontario — the heart surgery waiting list simply grew too long. The crack in the system was quickly papered over. It certainly wasn't the only such instance. In 1989, a report found that 24 British Columbians had died while waiting for heart surgery; a year earlier, a survey found that six heart patients had died in Manitoba's largest hospital waiting for the life-saving surgery (Goodman and Musgrave 516). All three provincial governments addressed the problem that had led to the untimely deaths. But there is a disturbing message here: every few years, the system falls so short that dozens of lives are lost.

Death from waiting is rare, but it does occur. Would this situation be acceptable in the private sector? What would happen if, on a routine basis, a handful of McDonald's customers dropped dead from eating spoiled beef?

1.4 Going South

"Was it difficult to leave?" rhetorically asks Dr. Robert Lifeso, a seventh-generation Canadian who practises in Buffalo, New York. "Of course. Two of my children were born there [in Canada]," he says with a hint of longing.

Lifeso graduated from medicine at the University of Toronto in 1969. After briefly practising in British Columbia and then abroad, in developing countries such as Nepal, he returned to school. He completed the orthopedic surgery residency and then received a fellowship in spinal surgery. He worked for the royal family of Saudi Arabia for a decade. In 1987, when his daughter was approaching school age, he decided to move back to Canada.

Lifeso wasn't happy with what he saw. "The bottom line was that governments [in Canada] weren't going to invest in hospitals or equipment — or health care." After weighing his options, he relocated to Buffalo. The decision wasn't easy, but the frustration of classmates who stayed in Canada helped to make it easier. "Either I went, or I could sit there and wish I was elsewhere."

Family experiences have also confirmed his darkest suspicions about the Canadian health care system. In the early 1990s, Lifeso's mother-in-law developed spinal stenosis. She was forced to wait eight months to see the necessary specialist, who wanted to run a diagnostic test. "At the time, MRI scans were extremely difficult to get in Toronto. Basically, no one got them." The alternative was a mylegram with a CT scan. "She was admitted to the hospital for the test. After, she ended up with terrible headaches. She was in the hospital for a week." Even with the confirmation, getting a surgeon was very difficult.

Lifeso decided to use his connections within the medical field. "I pressured a friend," he explains. "The surgeon was so busy, there was no post-op visit. She died in hospital of a pulmonary embolism [a fatal blood clot in the lungs]."

"The government has convinced people they have quality health care. It just ain't so, I'm afraid." So Lifeso practises within a 20-minute drive of the Canadian border. There, he believes, he has what it takes to practise medicine properly. When he does trauma surgery, he can get an MRI scan for a patient within 30 minutes. Nonurgent cases are scanned within 24 hours.

The necessities that Lifeso believes essential to a proper practice — high-tech equipment, hospital beds, and surgical theatres — are simply not available in his former home. "Canada has some of the best health care the 1970s can provide. But it's the turn of the millennium."

In an ironic twist, some of Lifeso's patients are Canadians who cross the border for better health care. Lifeso tells the story of a 69-year-old woman who is self-employed.

She has spinal stenosis. She can barely walk and is in a wheelchair.

Her son, a family physician, tried to get her in to see a spinal surgeon.

There are only two on the Niagara peninsula. The closest appointment would be . . . [six months away]. Her son begged the surgeon, "Please, it's my mother." "I don't care," the surgeon told him. "Everybody waits."

She explained to me that her quality of life is suffering. She doesn't want to wait until next year to get an appointment.

It's this sort of experience that leads the surgeon to a sharp conclusion: "When it comes to health care, Canada is just another third-world country. Scratch that," Lifeso insists. "Saudi Arabia is a bit better." He is careful to explain his views: "[I'm] not frustrated — disgusted is the word." When asked if he would return to Canada if conditions changed, there is no hesitation in his answer: "Absolutely. I would return to Toronto if I felt I could practise properly."

Dr. Robert Lifeso is not alone in his decision to leave Canada to practise elsewhere. In 1996, the Canadian Institute for Health Information reported that 713 physicians left the country — about the same number of physicians who graduated from five medical schools in Canada. The number marked roughly a 60% increase over the 1991 figure. But, in fact, this was an undercount. They only recorded the departures of physicians who practised in Canada before moving. Many of the young doctors opting for an American practice have never seen a single patient in Canada. In other words, the real exodus of physicians is considerably higher than indicated.

In 1995, writer Milan Korcok looked at the statistics from various family medicine programs across the country: "more than 33% of the University of Toronto's class of 1995 [is leaving the country], [along with] another 33% of the University of Alberta's last two classes . . ." ("Lost Generation" 895). In a recent study, Eva Ryten, the former research director at the Association of Canadian Medical Colleges, estimates that nearly half of the doctors who graduated in 1997 moved abroad. In 1991, only a third of new doctors left the country ("Brain Cramps").

There are many reasons why a physician may choose to leave the medicare system: the medical instability, the billing restrictions, the increasingly dictatorial nature of government. One of the strongest reasons is financial — the money is better south of the border. Young physicians with no job experience can be offered over $100,000 US as a starting salary. Given Canada's tax rates and provincial fee caps, no such opportunities exist north of the border.

Dr. Robert Harris, a plastic surgeon who specializes in hand and re-constructive surgery, is in the unusual position of practising in both Canada and the United States. A UBC medical graduate specially trained in both Canada and abroad, he practised in Montreal for 17 years. He then moved to Cornwall, Ontario. Today he practises there and just across the river — in Massena, New York.

His two practices are similar. Harris works in community hospitals in both countries, servicing communities of about 100,000 people each. As a result, he can accurately assess physician fees and incomes in the two countries: "There's no comparison. Fees are at least four times as much in the United States." For some procedures, Harris estimates that the fee gap is even higher: "Benign skin tumour — maybe 20 times as much." But major procedures, such as tendon surgery and rheumatoid hands, are four times as much, in US dollars. He adds that, given the conversion rate, "Right now that's five, six times as much." He continues down the list of procedures:

Debitron's disease: $300 in Ontario, $1,000 in the States — maybe twice that much depending on the insurance company. Breast reduction? In Ontario, $800. The lowest we are ever paid in the States is $2,500. Carpel tunnel in Ontario pays $144. In the States, $550.

Consultations and office visits do not have the same discrepancy. They would be more comparable. Consultation is $52.50 for my specialty in Ontario. The States: $75 US.

The answering service, telephone, electricity, office salaries are compa-rable. Taxes are not. In the US, there are many more things that you can claim. For example, you can write off one level's taxes against another. You can take municipal off state. In Canada, I take home about 20¢ for every dollar of gross income. In the States, about 34¢.

Of course, I give a bit more time to my American patients. Canadian patients have become accustomed to being rushed. It's a way of life in the Canadian system.

Harris isn't simply disappointed with the compensation. Like Lifeso, he finds that standards are far lower in Canada than in the United States: "We have the patients, [but] we can't process them. The patients pile up, and they just go on a waiting list. In the US, there's no shortage of operating room time. You can see them in the office one afternoon, then in the OR the next morning." For this and other reasons, Harris concludes that

The American patient gets a lot better care. When it comes down to the individual patient, Americans get more of the doctor's time and a better allocation of resources. I'd rather be a patient in the United States.

The non–life-threatening emergency — urgent cases — should get done in six to eight hours. Like a severed flexor tendon. According to the standards of the governing bodies of hand surgery, it should be treated in six to eight hours. In Canada, it will be done in three to four or five days. In Massena, the guy is usually up in the OR when I get there.

And in Canada patients are frequently bumped. "One weekend I saw a jaw fracture. He came in early Saturday morning after a car accident. I saw him around 8 a.m. I booked him before noon. I was bumped nine times. I wound up doing him Monday afternoon, just before dinner."

Harris goes on to summarize the differences between his two practices: "The big advantage over there is the ease with which I can get the work done there. I can process my patients. In Cornwall, I can't. There isn't OR time or bed space." He adds that,

> In Massena, I can treat my patients according to the textbook. In Canada, we are no longer practising to standard, and the gap between what we should be doing and what we are doing is growing. Now we are waiting a week to do cases that we had to wait 48 hours to do just a couple of years ago. These are cases we should do in a few hours.

It's just this frustration that caused surgeons such as Dr. Louis Pisters to leave the country. Featured in a front-page story in the *Globe and Mail*, he practises cutting-edge medicine with 14 other Canadians at the University of Texas–M.D. Anderson Cancer Center in Houston. The Texas hospital provides Pisters and his colleagues with the latest in diagnostic and surgical equipment, ample operating room time, and virtually unlimited research money (Abraham).

Physicians who have stayed in Canada aren't particularly happy either. They often complain about low morale. And government negotiations over fees have taken an ugly note lately. Although job disruptions by physicians were relatively rare in the past, they seem to be a monthly occurrence these days. Looking at the first seven months of 1998, we can draw up a long list of job actions. In fact, some or all of the physicians in five provinces were involved in some type of government protest. Doctors in both British Columbia and Quebec have staged large-scale, day-long work stoppages. Doctors in different parts of Alberta participated in some type of work disruption. In Manitoba, obstetricians announced their intention to engage in work disruptions, only to be bumped from the front page of the local paper in Brandon by the work stoppages of that city's physicians. Brandon physicians themselves were then bumped by Flin Flon physicians who briefly refused to perform even emergency surgeries.

It's not surprising that so many doctors would opt out — rather than put up with the instability and the confrontational environment, they choose to practise in another country. Of great concern is the number of talented physicians — particularly young ones — who are seeking greener medical pastures. Taxpayers should be troubled by the lost investment. A typical family physician has at least 10 years of university education, most of it in a heavily subsidized faculty of medicine. Based on conservative figures, each departing graduate in family medicine has had over $150,000 worth of educational expenses covered by taxpayers.[5]

But if taxpayers are saddened by the waste, they should be frightened by the implications of this exodus on health care delivery. In the short term, physician shortages wreak havoc on certain communities. The lack of anesthesiologists in Quebec, for example, has drawn public attention because surgeries have been cancelled and postponed. The shortage of endocrinologists (specialists of hormones and hormone diseases) in Saskatchewan has also caught the public's attention. In addition to these high-profile trouble spots, significant shortages of physicians in rural areas are common. In the long term, this trend will mean that the best doctors will systematically migrate south, leaving medicare with a shortage of talented physicians. And, given Canada's aging population (see chapter 5), this exodus will exacerbate a developing problem: the widespread shortage of physicians in Canada.

1.5 The Technology Gap

To the uninitiated, three months may seem like a long time. After all, it's the difference between the last warm days of summer and the first snowy days of winter, the difference between the heated and endless hours of a political campaign and the sweet honeymoon for the victor, the difference between a one-hit rock star's fame and his musical oblivion.

But to Dr. William Cavers, three months is a short time. Cavers, of course, isn't concerned about seasons, election campaigns, or rock stars. He worries about waiting times for MRI scans, and achieving a three-month wait for the patients of his Victoria practice has been a long, hard fight. A "victory," he declares with uncharacteristic enthusiasm. "It's fantastic, absolutely wonderful."

Victory may seem like an odd choice of words. But "war" was the word used by the BC minister of health to describe her interactions with Cavers and his colleagues. That a group of seven or eight doctors without so much as a listing in the phonebook arrived at such a bitter rhetorical battle with the BC government speaks volumes about the intellectual level of our health care debate.

What sparked this war? Victoria has only one MRI scanner, which is both funded and administered by the province. The waiting list to get a diagnostic test from the facility has ballooned in recent years. In October 1997, Dr. Darcy Lawrence, head of medical imaging for the Victoria area, raised the issue with the minister's staff. When nothing happened in the next four months, local doctors tried to raise the issue in early 1998 with the minister's staff through warlike efforts such as letter writing. After four months, the group decided to use the ultimate weapon of mass destruction: the fax machine. They issued a press release expressing their concern that waiting for MRI scans on Vancouver Island exceeded 11 months.

No doubt the public attention — and the doctors' promise to continue to draw public attention — caused Minister of Health Penny Priddy grief. But the real problem for her was not a handful of doctors and their fax machine but her government's lack of investment in high-tech equipment.

MRI scanners aid doctors in ways never thought possible. Just as the X-ray machine once revolutionized the world of diagnostic imaging, so too has the MRI scanner. But such equipment comes at a price — a high price. The machinery costs millions. A scan runs at $850.

Not surprisingly, then, British Columbia has relatively few scanners. With just one machine, Vancouver Island's facility serves 640,000 people. In contrast, the United States boasts a machine for every 50,000 people, and Europe has a machine for every 160,000 people (McArthur).

And, to the anger of doctors like Cavers, the government limited the number of scans performed at the facilities. At a time when patients were forced to wait over a year for the diagnostic test, the Victoria scanner was operating on bankers' hours, mandated to perform no more than 3,000 scans per year. Of course, ministry sources were quick to point out that patients in life-threatening situations can jump the queue and get scans quickly. Other patients were classified as getting "elective" scans.

But the term "elective" is deceptive. One patient on the waiting list, for example, was suspected of having an acoustic neuroma, a slow-growing cancer. For months, she waited, every day wondering if cancer was growing in her head. Patients suspected of having multiple sclerosis were also forced to wait. Imagine the sword of MS hanging over your head for a year. In an ironic twist, provincial regulations require that MS patients, in order to receive certain drug therapies, must have the disease confirmed first by an MRI scan.

The quality of health care available to other patients is also affected by such long waiting lists. Doctors who can't wait a year for MRI results are forced to choose painful, less effective tests. A neurosurgeon looking into nerve damage must perform a myelogram with a CT scan — instead of getting a simple MRI, patients with back injuries get a sharp needle in the spine and often develop a headache after the test. An ortho-pedic surgeon inspecting a bad knee will need to rely on arthroscopy — another painful procedure.

All this is what sparked the concern of Cavers. So he teamed up with other local doctors and formed the Victoria Physicians and Surgeons. Thus began a year-long journey through the many pitfalls of health care politics. Priddy eventually met with Cavers and his colleagues, even though she'd publicly said she wouldn't, yet she refused to address the group's concerns for months, even though she'd publicly said she would.

The final straw for the provincial government came when Mr. Kurchaba came forward. The BC resident had waited 11 months to get an MRI scan. By then, the tumour in his brain couldn't be removed without damaging his hearing in one ear. The long wait for an "elec-tive" test resulted in permanent hearing loss.

Priddy finally announced an increase in funding for MRI scans. As of March 1999, the waiting time for Vancouver Island sits at just over three months. For Cavers, this is a victory.

Problems with the availability of MRI scanners aren't confined to British Columbia. The province has nine scanners — about as many as Alberta, Saskatchewan, and Manitoba combined. Across the country, there are only 66 machines (Wickens 22). MRI scanners are scarce — there are more than eight times as many machines per person in the United States.

Many people are critical of comparisons with the United States, but, according to data obtained from the Winnipeg Hospital Authority, Canada doesn't fare much better when other international comparisons are made. In terms of the number of MRI scanners per capita, we rank behind Sweden, Britain, and South Korea. In fact, the list of countries with more scanners is impressively long: France, Austria, Spain, Switzerland, and Italy are all ahead of Canada. And such a comparison doesn't indicate the extent to which we have fallen behind. Austria, for example, has triple the number of machines per capita. Amazingly, Canada is on par with Latin American countries.

To put this problem in some perspective, consider that the Manitoba government has been excitedly touting the acquisition of a new MRI machine to help reduce waiting lists. And while the news has gathered local attention, the availability of MRI scanners is still depressingly inadequate. Currently, Manitoba has only 0.9 machines per million people. Even with the purchase, the province will have fewer MRI scanners per capita than the average for Latin American countries.

Far from being the exception, the lack of MRI machines is representative of the overall dearth of high-tech equipment available to Canadian patients. According to 1995 data, CT scanners — another diagnostic machine used to "see" soft tissue — are twice as common in the United States as in Canada. As part of the *Waiting Your Turn* study, the Fraser Institute surveyed doctors on diagnostic tests. Not surprisingly, doctors report long waits for many tests — an average wait of 9.6 weeks for an MRI scan, 4.1 weeks for a CT scan (Ramsay and Walker 18). A study that looked at waiting times for MRI scans at the two largest acute-care general hospitals in every larger city in North America found that Canadians tend to wait about 150 days for the procedure; by contrast, Americans wait only three days (Bell et al. 1015).

The lack of diagnostic equipment leads to unusual tales. In June 1998, *Maclean's* reported the strange story of Dr. Claude Nahmia (Wickens). Nahmia oversees the operation of two positron emission tomography scanners — diagnostic equipment that can produce cross-sectional images of cell activity to investigate various problems, including tumours, epileptic activity, and heart and brain functioning. In all of Canada, there are only seven such machines. They are so rare that Nahmia believes most physicians in nearby areas simply assume that the equipment he has isn't available to patients. For this reason, he brags about his short waiting period — usually less than two weeks.

1.6 The Valiant Defence

Medicare has its share of problems, but we should not overlook what we have. Compared with the vast majority of countries in the world, Canada has qualified and able physicians and nurses, decent hospitals, and a high level of care. The poorest of its citizens are not deprived of the care for lack of money, nor are the chronically ill.

Still, the problems facing our system cannot be overlooked. One way or another, they must be addressed — the status quo dooms us to a health care system with ever-increasing waiting lists, more talent slipping south, and a growing technology gap. The debate in Canada should be about how we resolve these issues. And yet, to a surprising degree, the so-called experts insist that many of the problems discussed in this chapter do not exist.

The Manitoba Centre for Health Policy and Evaluation is one of a handful of research centres studying the health care system. Like all such government-funded groups, the centre takes a rather uncritical view. A 1998 study on waiting lists is a case in point — although many people believe that waiting times for treatment are a problem, the centre is deaf to the reality. "Waiting Times Aren't That Long," screams the *Winnipeg Free Press* headline of the column describing the study by the centre (De Coster et al.). The study's authors find that waiting times for treatment are acceptable and, on a year-to-year basis, not increasing. The study also concludes that doctors who serve in both the private sector and the medicare system tend to make their medicare patients wait longer. The implications are twofold: medicare is working, and private medicine attempts to corrupt the public system.

The *Globe and Mail* dedicated more than a quarter of a page to the findings (see Coutts, "Cataract"). And when the Fraser Institute came out with its annual report on health care (which suggests that waiting times for treatment are long and continue to grow), the Manitoba study was used as a rebuttal. *The National* on CBC analysed the "methodology" of the Fraser Institute's work, and the *Globe and Mail* characterized it as "flawed" and "unscientific" (Coutts, "Patients").

In fact, it is the Manitoba study that deserves the criticism. Despite the sweeping conclusion that, "contrary to what is all-too-often reported, waiting times for surgery in this province [Manitoba] have remained stable," the government-supported group didn't look at waiting times across the system. The bulk of their work focused on only eight nonurgent surgical procedures, at least two of which are of questionable medical value. Dr. A.C. Harvey, head of the Department of Medicine at Misericordia Hospital in Winnipeg, states that, if the study had looked at high-demand surgeries, the findings would have been different. The wait for hip surgery, for example, has grown dramatically in recent years and, according to Harvey, was close to two years when the study was published.

In the study, the definition of waiting times is curious. The researchers measured the waiting period from the preoperative visit with the surgeon to the surgery. But this period represents only a part of the total waiting process — patients typically need to be diagnosed and then referred to a surgeon. Measuring waiting times for surgery in this way can be likened to judging an athlete's decathlon performance by her high jump. Anecdotal evidence and the Fraser Institute study suggest that the big bottlenecks in the health care system are getting an appointment with a specialist and getting high-tech diagnostic tests. The Manitoba study made no attempt to measure these waits.

And, in the one area where the Manitoba researchers looked at urgent surgery, the results hardly suggest that "waiting times aren't that long." Urgent heart bypass patients waited an average of four days for the surgery — a poor showing given that international standards state they should wait no longer than three days.

As for cataract surgeries, the study notes that waiting times have grown for the surgery over the past few years, though the authors are quick to point out that doctors who moonlight in the private sector have the longest waiting times for their patients. But what do the longer waits really mean? Some doctors are more popular than others; some have more operating room time than others. Time and popularity explain the difference in waits rather than a sinister influence of the private sector. Indeed, the comparison is hardly relevant. The question is not how waiting lists compare when private surgery is allowed; rather, the more pertinent questions to ask are "How long were the waiting lists before private surgery was allowed?" and "How long are the lists now?"

Even overlooking these problems, the Manitoba study isn't good news. It found that, after five years of provincial health reforms and increased government spending, waiting lists are not going away. The analytical problems and the ominous findings were not mentioned in the report.

The study, if dubious, is not an isolated example. Responding to an article in the *Winnipeg Free Press* suggesting that Winnipegers are concerned with their health care system, Manitoba Centre for Health Policy and Evaluation codirectors Charlyn Black and Noralou Roos denied that there are any problems. A lack of technology? "What types of technology? The evidence shows the number of Manitobans receiving several important procedures has actually increased since 1991, including cataract surgery (53 percent more) and hip and knee replacement (a 38 percent increase for hips and a 169 percent increase for knees)" (Black and Roos). An exodus of physicians? "On August 26, the *Free Press* published data from the Canadian Institute for Health Information showing that fewer physicians were leaving Canada . . ." (Black and Roos).

These statements aren't untrue, but they don't accurately represent the situation either. There are more hip and knee replacements performed in Manitoba now than in 1991, but because of an aging population waiting times have grown over the last half-decade. Access, after all, reflects not simply the supply of services but also the demand. And access to technology as measured in waiting for diagnostic tests has become worse in recent years. The Winnipeg-based Frontier Centre for Public Policy notes, for instance, waiting times for different tests in a recent article: four months for a CT scan, and six months for an MRI scan (Holle). It's also true to a point that fewer physicians are leaving Canada. Fewer left in 1997 than in 1996, but 1996 was a historic high. Only slightly lower than the 1996 figures, the data for 1997 were hardly encouraging. One could argue, using this logic, that Canada didn't have a deficit problem in 1986 because the deficit then was lower than in 1985 (a historic high).

The work done by the Manitoba Centre for Health Policy and Evaluation, then, reads like political spin, not like a substantive review of the data with appropriate conclusions. But it isn't the only group to interpret a mandate to study the system as a licence to defend it at all costs, even by denying the truth. Consider that, when the federal minister of health decided to investigate the waiting list issue in November 1997, he asked for a report from Health Canada. The government turned to six of the most prominent analysts in the field. After a year of study at a cost of $150,000, the researchers returned with a largely uncritical report suggesting that more information is needed. Indeed, the report took great pains to suggest that available data are "at best misleading . . . on access to care, and at worst instruments of misinformation, propaganda, and general mischief" (McDonald et al. ii).

For the most part, the experts are unmoved by the state of the medicare system. Whether it's waiting lists or the exodus of talented physicians, Canadians hear a startlingly uniform response from these experts: don't worry. Given the experiences of people such as Miriam Wiedman, Jean Gendron, and Twila Harris, it's not surprising that more and more Canadians are ignoring this "sage" advice. And with good reason.

2

The Sound of Silence

"SIR, WE HAVE the best health care system in the world." So responded Dr. Rey Pagtakhan to a hostile caller's question about waiting lists. Having established the superiority of medicare, Pagtakhan seemed to have little else to add, so the radio host moved on to the next caller.

Pagtakhan was once considered a rising star within the Liberal Party of Canada. As a physician from the North End of Winnipeg, he first ran for federal office in 1988. He was the sort of candidate the party's hierarchy liked: he had a professional background, was well known within the riding, and was prominent in his own (Filipino) community.

After a hard-fought campaign, Pagtakhan won Stanley Knowles's old seat and was off to Ottawa. Soon he became the Liberal health critic.

When Jean Chrétien announced his intention to seek the Liberal leadership in 1990, Pagtakhan was among the first to support the bid and was named one of two cochairs for Manitoba. All the cards seemed right for him to place highly within a Chrétien government. Rumours suggested that Chrétien had personally promised Pagtakhan the job of health minister before the election campaign of 1993. Here was the making of a perfect tale: an immigrant who works hard and becomes an important cabinet minister.

Somehow things didn't quite work out for Pagtakhan. When the dust settled, he wasn't given the health portfolio. Instead, Diane Marleau got the nod. Pagtakhan wasn't even named a minister. Years of hard work had failed to bear the fruit he had coveted. He was, however, given the chairmanship of a standing committee. Since then, he has largely concerned himself with employment equity and regulation of the Internet. He has seldom spoken in the House of Commons. A shuffle briefly made him parliamentary secretary to the prime minister. It's a far cry from running the Ministry of Health.

And so Dr. Rey Pagtakhan found himself on a radio talk show, in the fall of 1996, not as a cabinet minister but as a backbencher. But the callers didn't take pity on him.

After brushing aside the concerns about waiting lists, Pagtakhan answered the next caller, who wondered why he couldn't spend his own money on health care. Pagtakhan immediately replied, "as far as I'm concerned, there's no difference between the government spending money on health care and individuals spending money. The money is all coming from the same place: the taxpayer."

Another caller related a story about his experience waiting for treatment. A somewhat cross Pagtakhan immediately responded by criticizing the alternative: an American-style system in which the poor are on their own.

Thus went the morning — Pagtakhan defending the government's policies on medicare from an onslaught by critics. The comments were memorable because they were so unexceptional, so commonly heard. And that's the point.

Pagtakhan was challenged by numerous callers about the state of the health care system, and he offered nothing in reply but slogan after slogan. No matter what the concern, he avoided addressing it. The responses verged on the comical. His strategy — confuse the issue — mimicked that of the incompetent defence attorney on a bad TV movie: "Yes, you and your three friends saw my client hold the smoking gun as he fled the scene of the crime, but isn't it true that he was a decent neighbour?"

Just as Pagtakhan's performance was uninspired and unthoughtful, so too have been the comments made by practically every other active Canadian politician. This chapter explores the political debate on medicare.

2.1 The Health Care Script

Consider, for a moment, the actual arguments articulated by Pagtakhan and the questions that arise from them.

1. *Canada has the best health care system in the world.* Does Pagtakhan really believe this statement? How did he reach this conclusion? More importantly, does it somehow justify the problems within the system? Or does he believe that we have reached perfection?

2. *There is no difference between the taxpayer spending money and the government spending money.* Does Pagtakhan really not understand the difference between the state spending tax money and an individual purchasing goods and services? If there is no difference, why don't

we nationalize the clothing industry? Did the Soviet Union have an economy with the efficiency of that in the United States?

3. *The American system is the alternative — and we don't want that.* Is the only alternative to medicare an American-style system? Isn't it possible to create a better system without losing universality? Does Pagtakhan even understand the American system he so willingly vilifies?

This criticism may seem unusually sharp. Canadians have heard the above line so many times that the intellectual vacancy of Pagtakhan's position may be overlooked. But what if Pagtakhan provided similar arguments on another issue? Take rising youth violence in the inner-city as an example. If a caller phoned in with a disturbing story about her 10-year-old nephew being harassed and threatened by a gang, it's not difficult to imagine how a politician such as Pagtakhan would react. He would condemn the incident as unacceptable in our society. Then he would probably tout a possible solution to the problem of inner-city violence. He might even talk about addressing the roots of crime (the need for more job-creation and community-activity programs) or the punishment of crime (a call for stiffer sentences for gang-related violence and more police officers). But no politician would respond, "Sir, we have the safest streets in the world" or "Well, imagine how violent it would be if you lived in the United States." Such a dismissive, slogan-based response would be universally condemned. Yet, when it comes to medicare, Pagtakhan can offer exactly this type of response and not be held accountable by either his political colleagues or his constituents.

Pagtakhan has long been a defender of the status quo in health care. Perhaps this was why the Liberal government sent him in 1994 to London, England, to participate in the conference Health Care: International Comparisons. There Pagtakhan suggested that Canada is considered one of the best countries in the world "due to a large measure to its national health care system." Although the system faced rising costs, renewal would be possible without radical changes — "cost containment through improved efficiency of the delivery system." This renewal would be achieved, he suggested, by getting everyone involved in the process.

These comments are disappointing because Pagtakhan is an intelligent man. Having spent years as the Liberal health critic and, before that, as a physician, he must have greater insights on the matter. Even more disappointing is the fact that his comments on medicare are standard. His responses to legitimate concerns could be voiced by practically any politician today, provincial or federal. True, a New Democrat might throw in a line about corporate welfare, and a Reformer might discuss declining federal funding, but for the most part Canadians hear the same story about medicare from their federal politicians: the fundamental principles upon which the system rests are sound, and medicare is strong.

The extent to which politicians of all political stripes mouth the same slogans on medicare was well illustrated by a CBC Television debate on 26 May 1997, when *The National* hosted what should have been one of the most significant discussions of the federal election. A representative from each of the political parties was invited to debate the "Future of Medicare." Given the amount of attention the issue has gathered in recent years, it seemed like a timely opportunity for the different partisans to distinguish their visions for the social program. But the event was a dud — the political leaders had precious little to say.

All fundamentally believed in the system. All fundamentally recognized the importance of strong federal funding and national standards. All fundamentally opposed the concept of two-tiered medicine.

Sure, they had different ways of saying the same thing. The Progressive Conservative talked about a "health care guarantee"; the Reformer touted the importance of "prioritization so that we have money for health care"; the Liberal stressed "stable, long-term funding for health care"; and the New Democrat advocated "a strong national system." At the end of the debate, however, all were basically on the same page.

Let's recognize what the political partisans refused to acknowledge: medicare is in bad shape and will only get worse as the Canadian population grows older. Minor funding increases, politically motivated national standards, and meaningless guarantees aren't going to help much.

But an election campaign is rarely the time for detailed discussions of public policy issues. It is unfair to extrapolate general statements from the chaos and confusion of a five-week campaign. Let's therefore look in some detail at the two most important parties on today's federal political scene: the Liberal Party and the Reform Party. By analysing their positions on health care, we can indeed see that Canadian politicians are basically on the same page when medicare is discussed.

2.2 The Liberal Line

Being a centrist party has its advantages and its drawbacks. On the one hand, a centrist party is freed from the ideological constraints that its opponents on the left and right of the political spectrum must endure. If a particular policy is popular or practical, a centrist party can embrace it. There's no need to lose sleep over criticisms of inconsistency; it is hardly expected of so-called pragmatists. Thus, while the Reformers are expected to advocate less government all the time and the New Democrats are expected to advocate more government all the time, the Liberals are in the enviable position of being able to pick and choose. Unemployment insurance can be overhauled to make it more cost effective while taxes (or premiums) are raised for an unreformed Canada Pension Plan. There isn't even a pretence of consistency.

But, on the other hand, a centrist party is always threatened at both flanks. Adopting a particular policy born of compromise may alienate voters, losing them to the more ideological parties. Alternatively, failing to take a hard stand on a particular issue can also be troublesome. Many of the centrist parties in politics have been marginalized as a result. The Liberal Parties of Saskatchewan and Manitoba have suffered from this marginalization, as has their namesake in the United Kingdom. But the Liberal Party of Canada is able to maintain this constant and delicate balancing act, so Liberals have dominated the federal scene for most of the century. No wonder — the extent to which they capture the majority of the political spectrum is illustrated by the fact that there is a happy coexistence within the same cabinet of fiscal hawks, such as Paul Martin and John Manley, and leftists, such as Sheila Copps and Lloyd Axworthy.

With this frame of reference, it's easy to see why defence of the medicare system is such an important issue for the federal Liberal Party. The Liberals speak with great passion when they espouse this point of view. There's something ironic about the emotion — Liberals, after all, have hardly been an excitable lot in recent years. Instead, they have quietly prided themselves on "strong management." But when the issue of medicare surfaces, a transformation occurs. It's as though, having spent years watching other politicians get excited about issues, this is finally their turn. Yes, Preston Manning may have his "distinct society" position, and Lucien Bouchard may speak forcefully on sovereignty, but a passionate defence of medicare is for the Liberal Party.

Why the fuss? First, a vocal stand is popular with many Canadians. Medicare continues to poll well, even though the system may in fact be failing. An impassioned speech by the prime minister appeals to the majority of Canadians — even to supporters of other parties. On the right, some Reformers like the party's stand on tax cuts, deficit reduction, and the Constitution but are fearful of changes the party might make to the health care system. The Liberal Party suddenly offers a nice alternative. On the left, some New Democrats like the party's traditional role as the "social conscience" of Ottawa but find the claims of deficit reduction disingenuous. Again, the Liberal Party becomes a nice alternative. Medicare is a winning issue.

Second, defending medicare serves a useful role in holding the Liberal base together. Many party volunteers, donors, staffers, and even backbenchers hold political views that are left leaning. To them, the party's bid to oust the Progressive Conservatives in 1993 wasn't just about taking back power; it was also about doing things differently. Brian Mulroney's policies and initiatives, such as NAFTA, cuts to social programs, and a seemingly endless obsession with the deficit were all perceived to be perverse. The party's campaign theme of "jobs, jobs, jobs" symbolized the different approach. It was a call for an interventionist government that cared more about people than deficit figures, for a party that stood for job creation and national day care programs. But for these pink Liberals, Prime Minister Jean Chrétien's governance proved to be a rude awakening. NAFTA wasn't renegotiated. Paul Martin's budgets cut provincial transfers for health, education, and welfare much faster than Mulroney would ever have dared. And the deficit became the government's real obsession. The left Liberals wondered what had happened to the calls for more jobs and a national day care program.

Medicare is a social program that these Liberals hold close to their hearts. Medicare represents to them nostalgia for a past era when Liberals were able to do the compassionate thing and expand government without concern for deficits. By defending the program, the party's leadership is able to appease the left Liberals. It's a compromise of sorts: the fiscal hawks can balance the budget, but the lefties are assured that nothing will happen to the medicare system. It's not surprising that Chrétien chose a prominent left Liberal, Allan Rock, to be the minister of health but kept the fiscal hawks in charge of the financial portfolios.

Medicare, then, is more than a simple social program for the Liberal

Party of Canada. It is a glue that binds core Liberal supporters together. It is tempting to soft supporters of other parties. It is clever politics. Political handlers term this a "wedge issue" — polarizing yet popular.

Just how sincere, then, is Jean Chrétien's claim that he believes in medicare? Probably not very sincere. For all the rhetoric, the Liberals cut the transfer payments by $6 billion — a cut that certainly impacted on provincial medicare funding. This the prime minister allowed despite opposition from the Liberals on the House Standing Committee on Finance who urged the government to preserve transfer payments no matter what. And Chrétien has occasionally slipped. After the release of the 1995 budget, for example, he defended the transfer cuts by suggesting that his government wasn't wedded to the comprehensive and user fee-free design of the system. Originally, he noted, medicare was "intended merely to keep people from losing their homes" (qtd. in Feschuk).

The Five Principles

The Liberals chose to defend medicare in a selective way. With the fiscal hawks demanding and getting reductions to the transfer payments in order to achieve a balanced budget, it was clear that the Chrétien government wouldn't be financially defending the program. Instead, it chose a zero-cost method: the government has staunchly defended the status quo on the Canada Health Act. The position is well represented by the comments of David Dingwall, then the minister of health: "I don't mind debating the principles of the Canada Health Act, but those principles are just not negotiable."

The Liberal strategy has proven to be shrewd. Liberals can easily blame all problems with the medicare system on the provinces by pointing out that health care is, after all, a provincial responsibility, as set out by the Constitution. Thus, when a woman phones her local MP's office in Toronto to complain about the long wait for hip surgery, she is quickly given the phone number for Premier Mike Harris. Blame is thus deflected. But the federal government does have an important role as the guardian of the principles of medicare. So that woman isn't just sent away; she's first told how her Liberal MP is off fighting to ensure that the provinces aren't allowed to do more damage to the system. Political benefit is thus maximized.

The hard line on the Canada Health Act is not only the source of many speeches; the Liberals have to some degree also backed it in action.

Faced with growing waiting lists, an exodus of competent physicians, and declining quality of care, Alberta premier Ralph Klein did in 1995 what most provincial premiers had been thinking about doing for years — a little experimentation with the medicare system. Klein allowed semiprivate medical clinics to offer Albertans basic surgeries. Patients of these clinics were then charged a facility fee on top of the regular billing to the medicare system. Klein hoped that the clinics would help to lessen the burden on the public system and improve quality at zero cost. The move was bold and controversial. Unfortunately for the premier, the federal government also thought that it was dangerous. So, on 16 November 1995, the federal minister of health began docking Alberta transfer payments by $420,000 a month. By the spring, the experiment was over. Klein gave up.

Chrétien has made it clear that there is also to be no flexibility of the five principles of the Canada Health Act in the future. "When you have five conditions and you want to maintain them," he told reporters, "you don't give away the right of interpretation" (qtd. in Kennedy, "Liberals"). Thus responded the prime minister to the ongoing provincial demand that the provinces have a say in the interpretation of the Canada Health Act. In nonpolitical jargon: the provinces want flexibility in administration, but they're not going to get it.

The provinces have a legitimate grievance. The federal government contributes well under a quarter of the funds for medicare yet refuses to allow any flexibility. But this is really missing the point. The issue, after all, is more than a simple turf war between a domineering older brother and his smaller siblings. Medicare is in real trouble.

But, for the most part, the Liberals ignore this situation. Instead, they cling to the five principles of the Canada Health Act, which state that medicare is to have

1. *public administration* — administration and operation on a nonprofit basis controlled either directly or indirectly by the government;
2. *accessibility* — coverage without user fees by hospitals or extra billing by physicians (enforced by the threat of dollar-for-dollar financial penalties in transfer payments);
3. *comprehensiveness* — coverage for all "medically necessary" services;
4. *portability* — coverage for residents of one province in another province; and
5. *universality* — coverage for all residents of a province.

The irony is that, for all the Liberal rhetoric in defence of these principles, violations occur every day.

Portability should mean that a Quebecker getting medical care in Alberta wouldn't have to worry — the insurance coverage is portable. In fact, Quebec doesn't have an agreement with the other nine provinces. Many physicians in English Canada are reluctant to take Quebec patients because the Quebec government pays low compensation to physicians. And the Quebec government doesn't cover hospital stays in other provinces (Francis, "Ottawa"). Although the digression may seem minor, the result is unequivocal: the principle isn't upheld.

The principle of universality is supposed to mean that every citizen is covered by the state health insurance. But this isn't the case in several provinces where citizens are charged a small tax to help fund medical services. Those who don't pay that modest deductible are not, at least theoretically, covered by medicare. According to the BC Ministry of Health, approximately 97% of residents are covered — a full 100,000 people thus have no insurance in British Columbia (Ramsay, McArthur, and Walker 117). It seems that this isn't particularly consequential, because these residents are treated anyway, though several studies (like that of the Hull Commission) have suggested otherwise.

Even accessibility, it could be argued, doesn't truly exist. This is the principle that Canadians seem to hold most dear — that both princes and paupers will be treated equally by the health care system. Section 12.(1)(a) of the Canada Health Act (1984) clearly specifies that this must be the case — provinces must provide services with "uniform terms and conditions." But exactly how uniform are services when the waiting time for an MRI scan topped a year in Victoria yet pro basketball player Shareef Abdur-Rahim was able to jump ahead of 984 people to get a scan? (Kennedy, "Critical"). Uniform, that is, if you're not a Vancouver Grizzlies star.

In fact, medicare is not a one-tiered system in which every citizen is treated equally but a seven-tiered system. Some patients seem to be treated more equally than others. Consider the following comparisons.

- In terms of waiting lists, a patient requiring medical attention in Quebec receives more prompt care than one in Prince Edward Island (Ramsay and Walker, Waiting 23).
- Within provinces, the availability of care differs substantially, particularly between urban centres and rural areas. Kenora, Ontario, doesn't have a pediatric neurosurgeon within 200 kilometres. Toronto has several.

- Because Workers' Compensation Boards directly purchase health care, their clients receive treatment faster than other patients. This is an interesting situation. A man who falls down the stairs and injures his knee at work will get an MRI in four days; the same man, if he falls down a flight of stairs at home, will have to wait at least four months for the MRI (Bohuslawsky, "Politicians").
- Physicians use their connections to jump waiting lists for their own treatment. Dr. Grant Hill, the health critic of the Opposition, freely admitted this practice in a recent interview: "If I'm injured I don't go to the emergency room to sit there a long time and wait for somebody to see me" (qtd. in Chwialkowska).
- Preferential treatment for certain patients — particularly those with high public profiles or personal ties to treating physicians — is common. A survey of Ontario physicians by ICES found that 80% had been involved in the preferential care of a heart patient. And 53% of hospital executives had done likewise.
- The prime minister and the governor general are treated at the National Defence Medical Centre in Ottawa. Before 1994, the privilege included all federal politicians and senior civil servants.
- Canadians with the financial resources frequently go to the United States to purchase their health care. A clinic in Grafton, North Dakota (a short drive from the Canadian border), operates an MRI scanner, and 80% of the clientele is Canadian.

The infinite rhetoric about the five principles is hollow. But even if the federal government could enforce these principles, it would miss the point. We shouldn't judge the medicare system by these five principles, for doing so amounts to judging the success of a marriage by its ability to follow the prenuptial agreement — an easy but pointless exercise.

As the Liberals faced the campaign of 1997, polling suggested weakness on the medicare front. Yes, their role as the guardians of the system was popular, but Canadians had concerns. The horror stories reported in the media about the state of the system had convinced many that medicare was in trouble. The Liberals decided to take a more proactive role. Clearly, the five principles weren't negotiable, so there was relatively little room left in which to advocate meaningful reform. The task was further complicated by the federal government's insistence that health care administration was a provincial responsibility. This insistence meant that a package of intrusive initiatives was basically off the table. The Liberals were left in a position, then, to advocate only one option: the expansion of medicare.

Pharmacare

Imagine the New Democratic Party announcing a new social program to solve a problem that doesn't exist, and at the press conference leader Alexa McDonough admits that the New Democrats have no idea how much the program will cost or even how it will work. "We are working on that," she insists, "but it will save us money in the long run because government is more efficient than the private sector." Needless to say, the announcement would be greeted with scepticism. Commentators would quickly dismiss the proposal and remind us that the party is just trying to win votes from the left.

But what if the announcement were made by the Liberal Party? During the election campaign in 1997, Prime Minister Jean Chrétien addressed the Regina Chamber of Commerce. He used the opportunity to tout his party's commitment to a new social program, pharmacare. Asked about the cost, he replied, "we are working on that"; then he added that the party was determining "the extent of the program, the cost, [and] the savings" (qtd. in Greenspon, "Chrétien").

What the Liberals lacked in details they tried to compensate for in commitment. *Securing Our Future Together*, the Liberal platform (dubbed the Red Book II), tells us that the new Liberal government would "develop with [representative] groups a timetable and fiscal framework for the implementation of universal public coverage for medically necessary prescription drugs" (75). Prescription drugs would be covered under the Canada Health Act. The proposal was bold, ambitious, and utterly pointless. Perhaps this was why commentators didn't take it seriously, but they should have, for it speaks volumes about the Liberals and their inability to address the fundamental problems with medicare.

The Liberals seem to be sold on pharmacare, but should they be? The public sector's role in the payment of pharmaceuticals is already sizeable, amounting to 32% of total expenditures. Medicare covers all drugs administered during institutional care, including hospital stays. And every province already has a program in place to cover prescription drugs for the poorest citizens. Those who need government-funded drug coverage have it.

The rest of us are doing just fine. Most Canadians are covered by an employer-funded or private drug insurance; only 12% of Canadians have no insurance, and there's no evidence to suggest that they require any government help. Most of the uninsured are young and healthy citizens who figure that the limited benefits of insurance are outweighed by the costs.

A national pharmacare program is unnecessary, but politicians will be politicians. Thus, the Liberals proposed not only to cover the 12% who are uninsured but also to introduce a national program to pay for the prescription drugs of every Canadian.

The cost would be tremendous. Canadians spend about $6.5 billion a year on prescription drugs. Even a national version of the BC pharmacare plan would be about $4 billion per year, and such a plan would be unacceptable to the Liberals because its deductibles, limitations on drug coverage, and reliance on private insurance conflict with the Canada Health Act.

The Red Book II insists that government coverage would be cheaper than the current system because administrative expenses are reduced in a public system. This is doubtful. Although some expenses may be lower, overall costs are likely to be much higher. Government isn't efficient. More importantly, in a "free" system people consume more. Consider a young man with a strained back. His doctor gives him a physical, concludes that there's no serious injury, and prescribes a strong painkiller. A choice must be made: is the pain great enough to warrant the expense of the prescription, or will a couple of aspirins do the trick? With pharmacare, there's no decision to be made — the drugs are free.

Demand unchecked by cost means a dramatic rise in expenditures because consumers have no incentive to economize. The British government discovered this problem when it experimented with "free" drugs in the 1960s. After three years, modest user fees were reintroduced, and demand fell by 30% over six months. Even Communist Hungary eventually implemented user fees for prescription drugs after the government recognized that not every comrade was interested in the common good.

It seems, then, that a pharmacare program would inevitably lead to the rationing of prescription drugs as the government scrambles to limit the surge in demand. Health economist Cynthia Ramsay suggested to me that "A national pharmacare program will only bring rising costs and reduced access."

Despite all the evidence, the Liberals stood by their promise, insisting that full public funding of prescription drugs was a recommendation of the National Forum on Health. True, but hardly convincing, for the forum's credibility is dubious at best. The final report of the government-appointed committee ignores even the most obvious problems with the medicare system. Such a report should hardly be taken seriously.

Some observers doubt that pharmacare will ever see the light of day, believing that it was merely election talk. For the moment, pharmacare is dead. More than two years after the Liberal reelection, it is a forgotten whisper from a distant campaign. A lack of provincial support coupled with the high costs of such a program has left the Liberals to tout their commitment to medicare in another way — with "reinvestment." Of course, with surpluses as far as the eye can see, pharmacare may one day be resurrected in a yearning to spend. For the time being, the Liberals have settled on a different strategy for medicare: increasing its federal funding in the "health care" budget.

Whether the approach is to expand medicare with pharmacare or to sink more federal money into an unreformed ailing system, the Liberal Party has established itself as the party of health care status quo. At a time when the house is on fire, the Liberals have busily talked up the prospect of building a garage and then finally settled on renovating the kitchen. The needed discussion on alternatives to the failing system is taboo. Ironically, the party that touts itself as the great defender of medicare has thus ensured its inevitable failure.

2.3 The Reform Party

"It's a lie!" replied Dr. Grant Hill's assistant to the suggestion by some people that his party supports two-tiered health care (telephone interview, 9 June 1997). "The party has never supported two-tier medicine," he added with equal emotion. The response was sharp but not unexpected. The Reform Party has spent a considerable amount of time and energy attempting to distance itself from any suggestion of support for two-tiered medicine.

The staffer then went back to the script that Reformers would like people to remember: the Liberal Party has cut medicare, while the Reform Party believes in more funding. "It's an underfunded, badly managed program," the staffer explained, "and the Reform Party thinks it's higher priority than canoe museums in [Chrétien's riding of] Shawinigan."

This was the line often used by the Reform Party in the 1997 election campaign. With no hint of new ideas or alternative funding mechanisms, the party found a popular — and, it hoped, winning — strategy on medicare: by talking about the need to increase funding, the Reformers could criticize the Liberals, emphasize their commitment to health care, and, most importantly, talk about medicare without really talking about it. Reform's platform, *A Fresh Start for Canadians*, reflected the strategy. It scarcely mentioned medicare and contained only one promise for the program:

> The federal government's share of funding for Canada's Medicare system has been falling for two decades. The result has been a funding crisis that has led to hospital closures, growing waiting lists, and declining national standards. To this end, a Reform Government will increase federal funding for Health Care. A total of $4 billion each year in additional federal funds will be injected into Health Care and Post-Secondary Education. (Reform Party of Canada 18)

In fact, the pledge wasn't nearly as generous as it seemed. The platform also stated that funding to welfare would be cut by $3.5 billion a year. The provincial transfer (the Canadian Health and Social Transfer), which covers health, education, and welfare, would thus be increased by $4 billion for health but cut by $3.5 billion for welfare. As David Frum noted, "They [Reformers] are hoping Canadians will not notice that these two promises cancel each other out" ("Reform"). From a provincial point of view, then, the offer was hardly amazing. The Reform Party promised to give with the right hand and to take with the left hand.

It is significant, though, that the Reform Party chose such a strategy walking into the 1997 election. Not that long ago, Reformers did say more about medicare. In fact, over the years, the party has held various positions on the issue. For this reason, perhaps, the doubts about Reform and two-tiered health care persist.

Position 1, 1987–92

In the early years, the Reform Party suggested that the way to save medicare was to return it to its original role: that is, to help the needy pay for medical bills, while others would face various forms of payment. The implementation of such changes would be left up to the provinces.

At the founding convention, Reform Party delegates were vague on medicare, agreeing only that "adequate health insurances are available to every Canadian." In August 1988, delegates to the party's policy convention approved several election planks, including a call to end the universality of medicare. In a postconvention interview, Preston Manning suggested that ending universality would help to make the program more financially viable and available for the needy (Barnett). The logic was straightforward: "If someone tells you the government can pay 100 per cent of the costs of 100 per cent of the services for 100 per cent of the people, then they are misleading you," Manning said in a later interview (qtd. in Winsor).

During this period, Manning spoke often about the ability to pay. The financial reach of Widow Smith and Peter Pocklington differs, Manning argued, so their share of payment should also differ (Winsor). He made it clear that the widow should always be assisted by the state. People like Pocklington were a different matter. User fees and insurance premiums were inevitable to keep medicare from dying.

The actual reform of health care would take place at the provincial level. The Reform Party advocated loosening up the Canada Health Act to allow provincial experimentation. Provinces would then be able to try user fees, premiums, and copayments. Manning didn't believe that it was the federal government's role to determine which income levels would have to pay what percentages of cost. "Administration" was left to the provinces. The Reform Party's goal was simply to provide the provinces with a workable framework.

Position 2, 1993

When the 1993 election campaign drew closer, the party line softened. By campaign's end, Manning seemed to back away from his earlier position.

In the crucial days just before and during the campaign of 1993, when the Reform Party would be transformed from a little-known western party into a national political force, Manning said little on health care. The Reform Party's position was promoted as a simple extension of its popular line on balancing the budget: deficit spending results in higher debt-servicing charges that draw money away from social programs. In a news release, "Out of Control Government Spending Killing Medicare," Manning was clear: "The real threat to health care is out-of-control federal spending and a lack of social spending priorities." The message was fiscally conservative and popular, but it didn't really address the growing problem with the medicare system. During the campaign, Manning did speak about "flexibility," but the dominant health care theme was essentially about balancing the budget. Not surprisingly, the *Calgary Herald* ran an article at that time titled "Health Care: Even Canada's Most Fiscally Conservative Politicians Know They Mess with Medicare at Their Peril" (see Toneguzzi).

As the party's popularity surged, criticism from the traditional parties became more serious and focused on Reform's health care policy. NDP leader Audrey McLaughlin charged that Reformers would leave Canada with an "Americanized" health care system (qtd. in Wilson-Smith 17). Jean Chrétien also suggested that "the rich will have a very good system" while "the poor will have nothing" (qtd. in Wilson-Smith 18). The criticism threatened to hurt the Reform Party. Asked in a radio interview if he supported user fees, Manning gave an unequivocal — and surprisingly inconsistent — answer: "No, we don't and we never have. And this idea that we've promoted U.S.-style health care or user fees or deductibles is fundamentally false" (qtd. in Ferguson).

Position 3, 1994–96

After the surprisingly strong election result, Reformers again talked freely about changing the nature of medicare by devolving power to the provinces and then deinsuring services.

Manning spent much time advocating a decentralization of medicare. Allowing the provinces to decide how to administer the program, he said, would give them a flexibility in administration that could save it. His comments in a 1994 address to the Ontario Hospital Association summarized the position:

> Loosening the Canada Health Act would give provinces other options besides closing hospitals and rationing health care. It would enable them to experiment with options such as user fees, deductibles, and private delivery of services, if they choose to do so, without fear of punishment by the federal government, so long as universal access to the health care system is assured. ("Health Care Reform")

The position was similar to the old Reform Party line: leave medicare up to the provinces so that they can experiment with it. But Manning stopped short of his original assessment. User fees and coinsurance were no longer absolutely necessary for the survival of the system, but such options would facilitate a more efficient system. And he didn't endorse a two-tiered medicare system. It isn't wrong to assume that such changes could give rise to a privately funded system in addition to a publicly funded one. Manning, however, was careful to distance himself from such a position — it would be up to the provinces to make such "administrative" decisions. If the government of, say, Nova Scotia were to allow private insurance and private clinics, it would be up to the voters in that province to hold their government accountable.

In 1995, the Reform Party began advocating the idea of deinsuring certain services. In Saskatchewan, Manning called for a national debate on the topic. Dr. Grant Hill, Reform's health critic and a physician, outlined the position frequently and articulately: core services should be funded, others not. Patients would thus be required to pay for noncore services and, if they so chose, privately delivered core services. His "Medicare Plus" position was the topic of speeches, newsletters, and even an article in the *Globe and Mail*. "Canadians must have health care choices," he declared. A Reform bill was debated in the House of Commons. "These reforms," Manning explained, "are required to preserve the best features of the present system" (qtd. in Menzies).

As much as Manning danced around the issue, preferring to speak to the Ontario Hospital Association about "provincial flexibility" to better health care, his MPs were bolder. Dr. Keith Martin, a physician, was blunt: "we need to amend the Canada Health Act to allow for private clinics and services, where only private moneys are exchanged," he wrote in a letter to the Canadian Medical Association on 12 March 1996. He continued:

> Some would argue that doing this would produce a better private system than the public one and this is probably true. . . . But is it not better to have an unequal system that provides for better access for all people rather than the current system that is providing for rapidly declining access for almost everyone?

Position 4, 1997

As discussed above, the Reform Party avoided making any comments on controversial issues, such as user fees, and instead emphasized the need for more funding.

All the talk of "choice" and "provincial flexibility" ended as the 1997 election campaign approached. Preston Manning changed the tune: more money for health care was the important thing. As well, he repeatedly stated that strong national standards comprised one of the federal government's 10 roles. Even Dr. Grant Hill abandoned his hard stance on two-tiered health. Although he argued that the government should "Europeanize" medicare — that is, allow a parallel private system — in an interview just before the election (see Sullivan), he made a very different argument during the debate about medicare on CBC's *The National* a few weeks later (26 May 1997): "Two tier is not on in Canada at this point in time. Put the money back in medicare and I think this argument will be pushed away."

There is, then, some justification for the scepticism of Reform's health care position: it has hardly been clear over the years and certainly not consistent. And while the party may officially shun the idea of two-tiered health care, it has at least flirted with the idea in the past, and some MPs have clearly endorsed it.

In all fairness, the criticism of Reform should be taken in context. Holding politicians to their stated positions is like trying to keep a grip on a fish. Political parties have a habit of squirming their way from one position to another on key issues. Pierre Trudeau mocked his Conservative opponent for promising to implement a temporary freeze on wages and prices and then did just that after being elected; the Progressive Conservatives under Brian Mulroney were elected on a platform of balancing the budget and then proceeded to triple the debt; Jean Chrétien and his party promised to renegotiate NAFTA or abrogate — they did neither and then became passionate free traders. Parties' ideological stands must be tempered by the reality of governance.

But the Reform Party's position hasn't been corrupted by days in office, for the party has never governed. And while comparisons to other parties are useful, they are deceptive — Reform isn't like a traditional party. It has a history of taking controversial issues, such as deficit reduction, and drawing up detailed plans. It even goes one step further and tells voters that, if Reformers do not live up to their promises, they can be held accountable by a recall vote. And the party "guarantees" the platform in *A Fresh Start* (1).

Why is it that a party with such clear views on spending and taxes can't advocate a clear message on health care? University of Calgary Professor Tom Flanagan, author of *Waiting for the Wave: The Reform Party and Preston Manning*, and former Reform Party director of research, suggests political pragmatism. "My impression," he said during a phone interview, "is that they have backed away from confronting the system in any way." Flanagan speculates that many within the party would support "more market-orientated competition" but that they have been "beaten up quite badly in previous years over the issue." For this reason, "internally they could not agree on how to sell [change]."

Not even the Reform Party is willing to advocate real changes to the medicare system and stick to the message. As Flanagan observed, "the position is not nearly so much of a challenge to the status quo as the party has done on other issues." This last point is particularly important. Consider how many controversial positions the Reform Party advocated in its 1997 election platform:

- privatization of the Canada Pension Plan;
- billions of dollars in cuts to the federal government;
- termination of thousands of civil service positions; and
- privatization of CBC Television, Via Rail, and Canada Post.

As simple as the issue is for the Liberal Party, the federal government's role in reforming medicare is a difficult issue for the Reform Party. On the one hand, party members are pulled by their ideological instincts — conservatives believe that a public system is inefficient and ineffective. Moreover, individuals should be allowed to spend their money as they please. For this reason, the party should naturally prefer two-tiered medicare and other free-market alternatives to the present system. But, on the other hand, the party has a strong populist streak. Yes, Reform is about smaller government, but it's also about MP recalls, free votes in the House of Commons, and other initiatives that move political decision making closer to the people. How, then, can the party support a program so unpopular with the Canadian people? And, if the Prairie populist instincts aren't strong enough, perhaps the desire for electability is. Reformers, after all, want to get elected.

Hence, the Reform Party entered the election campaign of 1997 with a strategy that attempted to out-Liberal the Liberals: more funding coupled with strong national standards. The party strategists clearly decided that, if they couldn't beat the Liberals on unreformed medicare, they shouldn't just join them — they should pull to the left of them. The approach was not only wrong in light of the real problems facing the system but also embarrassingly inconsistent with the overall direction of the party.

In a particularly biting editorial, the *Ottawa Citizen* summarized the Reform position on health care:

> Reform wants less federal spending in general, but more on the Canada Health and Social Transfer. . . . It respects provincial autonomy, favours national standards in health, wants to broker a deal with the provinces on these standards, wants more money spent on transfers for health, and opposes federal financial intrusions in areas reserved to the provinces by the Constitution, like health. ("United Non-Alternative")

The contradictory positions on health care over the years reflect this internal struggle between ideology and electability, conservatism and populism. On medicare, Reform at once supports decentralization and strong national standards, no user fees and provincial flexibility that could introduce user fees, more health care funding and decreases to the provincial transfers that essentially offset the higher funding.

And since the election, the Reform Party has worked hard to establish itself as the party of more money for medicare. In the 1999 prebudget submission, finance critic Monte Solberg wrote: "because the Liberal government made a deliberate decision to slash $16.5 billion (cumulative) in health transfers, 188,000 sick people are right now on hospital waiting lists" (Reform Party of Canada 3). His plan promised to end the "siege by Ottawa" (6) and put $2 billion immediately into medicare. Even though the federal budget bested Reform's proposal, Manning attacked the government: "The real result . . . is a two-tiered health-care policy where ordinary Canadians get put on a list 200,000 names long and wealthy Canadians go to the United States. My question to the Prime Minister is how does it feel to go down in history as the father of two-tiered health care?" (qtd. in McCarthy).

If there has ever been a party that has "challenged the status quo," it is the Reform Party. Born as a western rebellion against the Mulroney government, Reform has been controversial since its founding convention. In 1992, for example, the party opposed the Charlottetown Accord, a compromise supported not only by the ruling Progressive Conservatives but also by both opposition parties in the House of Commons and by the provincial premiers. That practically all politicians in the national picture endorsed the deal didn't phase Reformers. Their bold stance paid off — the accord bombed in a referendum on the issue, and the Reform Party gained immeasurable credibility.

But health care is a different matter. Reform has discovered the hard way that there is no benefit in speaking the truth about the medicare system. Yes, waiting lists are long and continue to grow, quality physicians are moving to greener pastures across the border in record numbers, and the aging of our population ensures that the system will get much worse with time. But advocating changes in medicare is a thankless task. Indeed, it's a recipe for disaster. Critics are quick to play the "America card" — that is, the charge that changes will lead to an Americanization of medicare. And Reform doesn't want to deal with that.

Such a gutless approach illustrates the absolute fear politicians have of the issue. Not even the party that represents a rebellion against "Ottawa thinking" (support for multiculturalism, open immigration, bilingualism, high taxes, distinct society status), not even this group of fearless antiestablishmentarians, can say anything meaningful on health care.

The badly needed national debate on the issue isn't taking place. There is only the sound of silence as partisans of every political stripe advocate the intellectually vacant position of maintaining the status quo in an ideal system that doesn't really exist.

2.4 Why the Silence?

Surely the problems with our medicare system merit a response. When violent crime increases, politicians pledge action. Task forces mull the causes of and propose solutions for high unemployment. As the Quebec issue unfolds, academics propose differing but dramatic answers. The big issues of our time — crime, unemployment, Quebec — are the sources of infinite analysis and contemplation. But as our health care system worsens, not much happens. Even think tanks — those organizations expected to tackle the pressing issues of the day — tend to avoid this issue. The C.D. Howe Institute, for instance, hasn't turned out a single paper or book on the topic in the last four years, despite an impressive publication rate on subjects ranging from monetary policy to welfare. (The Fraser Institute is an exception to this rule.) Why is the state of the health care system so different from these other political issues?

Medicare is a *very sensitive issue*. More important, certainly, than any other issue. After all, most government programs affect a small portion of the population at any one time. Consider, for example, the subsidization of university education. Although billions of dollars are spent each year on our country's universities, many young Canadians never get degrees. And those who do tend to think little about their alma maters upon graduation. As a result, higher-education reform is contentious only to those directly involved in the system: professors, support staff, and administrators (the "new class," according to Irving Kristol).

Medicare is a different matter because in time we all get sick. Almost every citizen is touched by this government program. It's partly for this reason that voters are so sensitive to provincial health reforms. Unlike changes to the university system or art funding, changes to medicare affect — and possibly threaten — each citizen. The amalgamation of two graduate programs at the University of Toronto or cutbacks to an art gallery that displays paintings designed to shock the bourgeois don't capture the attention of a nervous public. The closing of an emergency room or any other decision that may affect the quality and availability of care for a community — that is, for you and your family — is another matter entirely.

Of course, this explanation is only partially satisfactory. Most people are concerned about crime, yet politicians advocate different strategies to combat it.

So what makes medicare unique? It has become a sacred trust — politically, it is beyond discussion. Even provincial politicians, such as Ralph Klein, who have cut funding and advocated changes still swear that they oppose major changes such as full two-tiered health care (see Menzies). An American journalist described a speech delivered at a fundraising dinner by Ontario premier Mike Harris: "For forty-five minutes, it was unabashed Reaganism. Then health care came up. Suddenly, I was in Sweden."

Why the silence? There are several possible explanations.

First, while medicare may mean different things to different people, most Canadians associate it with health care. For a high school student from suburban Toronto, medicare is an X-ray after a hard tackle on the football field. A middle-aged woman from urban Vancouver, on the other hand, sees medicare as an annual breast examination on which she insists because her mother died of breast cancer. And an elderly man from rural Nova Scotia understands medicare to be the life-saving cancer treatment he requires. But for all these people, medicare is equated with health care.

There is a difference between the two. Medicare isn't health care; rather, it's a funding mechanism. But because the two concepts are confused by many, medicare over the years has become viewed as the only way to achieve quality, accessible health care.

Second, Canadian experts uniformly back medicare. Health economists and policy analysts swear by the system. Rachlis, Decter, Deber, Evans, and Kushner may not be household names, but they are the ones quoted by the media when a health care issue arises. And whether it's a panel discussion on *The National* or an analysis by Jane Coutts in the *Globe and Mail*, these experts back the medicare system fully. They serve as the chorus to which the insistence of politicians is credible.

Third, the face of medicare that most Canadians see — that is, the primary care provider — has been relatively untouched by the problems with the system. Although long waiting lists exist for most surgical procedures and diagnostic equipment is in short supply, the family doctor is readily available.

Fourth, perhaps the strongest reason why medicare is untouchable stems from its initial success. For the better part of two decades, Canadians, regardless of socioeconomic status, enjoyed quality, "free" health care. In fact, medicare was a source of national pride. Politicians from around the world marvelled at the effectiveness of the program. Perhaps most flattering of all was the praise medicare drew from some American sources — although Canadians were hopelessly overshadowed by American sporting successes in the Olympics, American military might overseas, and American business empires that spread across the land, health care was something that we did better. Medicare, in short, was more than a simple funding mechanism — it became a source of national pride.

Unfortunately, though, the factors that contributed to medicare's initial success have long since changed. When medicare was introduced,

- half the population was under the age of 21, placing a light load on the health care system;
- the country enjoyed a booming economy that was rapidly growing;
- the government borrowed heavily to meet its financial obligations; and
- the "high-tech, high-expense" medical revolution hadn't yet started.

Three decades later, not one of these four factors holds. The boom years are over — our growth rate is stable and respectable but sluggish compared with that of the 1960s. Canada's demographics have shifted and are continuing to do so: the ratio of taxpayers to seniors is shrinking, meaning that more people are utilizing the system and proportionately fewer people are paying for it. In addition, tax dollars once available for health, education, and other programs are needed to finance the nation's large debt. And technological and pharmaceutical advances in the field of medicine have resulted in new financial burdens on the system.

By and large, Canadians don't see these changes. Medicare is perceived to be the only way to deliver health care. It was no surprise, then, that Reform Party leader Preston Manning tried to make health care funding a major issue during the 1997 campaign by charging that the prime minister was the "Dr. Kevorkian of the medicare system" (qtd. in Gray, "Health Care" 57). Or that Prime Minister Jean Chrétien distanced himself from provincial hospital cuts in a year-end interview with *Maclean's*, just months before the 1997 election.

Canadian politicians refuse to consider true reform of medicare for one simple reason: the program is popular but fatally flawed, and nobody wants to be the first to say so.

3

Health Care South of the Border

A number of months ago, a local TV station ran a news report comparing two families — the kind of human-interest story that fills time on a typical slow news day: one family lives in Kansas, the other in Saskatchewan. Despite the difference in citizenship, the two families have relatively similar lives — the men work in blue-collar jobs, the women tend to the children, and the kids are overly interested in their Nintendos.

But when health care comes up, the Americans seem to live in a different world. When the American husband falls ill, he gets the care he needs, but his hospital bill exceeds $60,000. Imagine the burden this amount places on his family.

In Canada (the report suggests) we just don't appreciate what we have. We complain often about problems with the health care system, but how many of us stop and consider the alternative? The alternative, of course, is an American-style system. But looking at that system of private health care, it's difficult to tell why we would want to abandon our medicare. The American system costs vastly more for users, yet millions of Americans are uninsured. Yes, some have better care, but 40 million poor Americans are deprived of even basic health care.

Canadians should take heart — when it comes to health care, we've got it right. By leaving health care up to the private sector, Americans have created a terrible system riddled with high administrative costs (resulting in expensive care), endless red tape, and many uninsured people.

*   *   *

Canadians often hear such stories that compare our "compassionate" medicare with the "heartless" American health care system. These stories like to emphasize what we all believe about the US system: that it is largely private with little government involvement, that the poor are often uninsured and without proper care, and that the administrative costs are high and unavoidable.

None of these beliefs is true.

Americans, it turns out, don't really pay for their health care. The American family in the above story, for instance, wasn't actually responsible for paying the $60,000 bill — their insurance company was. This misconception is typical. Canadians consistently view the American system as being completely "private." In fact, federal and state governments play a huge role in both the regulation of the health care industry and its financing. And — perhaps most surprisingly of all — the root problem with the American health care system isn't that different from medicare's flaw.

3.1 The Joke

A young woman visits a psychiatrist for the first time. To begin the session, the doctor recommends that they look at some ink blots. Pulling out the first nondescript picture, he asks her, "What do you see?"

She replies without hesitation, "Sex!"

The psychiatrist is surprised but, being a professional, simply nods and pulls out the next ink blot. "And now?"

Again, without hesitation, she says, "Sex!"

Showing her a third picture, he asks, "And this time?"

"Sex!"

After a moment of thought, the psychiatrist says firmly, "I think you have some problems we need to discuss."

"I have problems?" the woman asks. "You're the one showing all the dirty pictures."

The joke isn't unlike our dialogue on medicare. No matter what aspect of medicare is being discussed (alternative funding mechanisms, provincial jurisdiction, home care, deinsurance of noncore services, new technology), the conversation inevitably drifts toward the American health care system.

That the US system is mentioned on occasion in our discussions about medicare is hardly surprising. The United States, after all, is our neighbour and largest trading partner. Hence, comparisons with the United States often serve as points of reference in other public policy debates about taxes, trade, and crime. But the state of the American health care system isn't merely a point of reference in our ongoing debate about medicare; it's also a source of infinite analysis verging on obsession.

The typical panel discussion on "the future of health care" features two experts who become deeply engrossed in a technical dialogue about various provincial reform efforts, statistical trends, and insider observations. One panelist will then throw out the idea of user fees. A big mistake — he is quickly attacked by his counterpart. "User fees will cause an Americanization of medicare," he is told sharply.

The charge is weighty, and the response is always defensive: the accusation is denied, or the original idea is watered down. This exchange happens so often that Canadians rarely stop to ponder the full meaning of the accusation. What is this Americanization we so fear? What does it mean?

And while little thought has been given to these questions, the fear of Americanization has seeped into the national psyche, profoundly influencing our public policies and politics. Writing in the *Wall Street Journal*, Washington editor Albert R. Hunt calls health care "the defining political issue of the 1990s [in the United States]. . . . More than the economy or war and peace or abortion, this issue persistently arouses America's passions. It has shaped and reshaped the body politic throughout the decade." These words aptly describe the Canadian political scene. The irony is that it's the American health care system — or, more correctly, Canadian perceptions of that system — that has so shaped and reshaped our body politic.

Consider, for example, the power of the cry of "Americanization!" during the last federal election in Canada. In the dying days of the 1997 campaign, the Liberal Party was concerned that the strength of the Reform Party in the west would cost Liberals a majority government. When the election was called in late April, the Reform Party was weak. Polling had pegged its support far below 1993 levels. Liberal Party strategists assumed that the Liberals would thus pick up seats in the west — enough to compensate for losses sure to come as the New Democrats and the Tories enjoyed a resurgence in popularity.

Election campaigns are unpredictable, and the Reform Party soon gained ground. By midcampaign, it was clear that Preston Manning was doing very well in the west. Political analysts were beginning to talk of Official Opposition status. Liberal strategists became quite concerned and set out to find a way to break their opponent's electoral lock on Alberta and British Columbia. The Reform Party's stands on taxes and national unity were popular, but health care, Liberals hoped, would be another matter. Thus, for two weeks, Liberals aired ads attacking Manning's stand on medicare.

One of the TV attack ads was simple and to the point. After reading comments made by Manning, a male voice explained that the ideas "sound like American-style health care . . . and could cost as much." The basis of the ad was shaky at best. For all the Liberals' rhetorical support for medicare, their record was very different — provincial transfers for health, education, and welfare had been cut by a third over their term in office. And it wasn't as though the Conservatives or the Reformers advocated substantial changes to health care. In fact, both right-wing parties spent much time and energy trying to convince Canadians that they would out-Liberal the Liberals by increasing funding to medicare while enforcing strong national standards.

Even Manning's supposedly controversial statements were misleading. Yes, Manning had advocated provincial experimentation, but that was back in 1994. In 1997, he was a born-again believer in medicare, and his strongest criticism of the campaign came when he accused the prime minister of being the Jack Kevorkian of medicare because of funding cuts. There was further irony in the attack ads. In the 1994 speech, Manning himself had participated in some American bashing when talking about his vision for medicare.

But the Liberals hoped that Canadians would overlook these points and focus instead on the potential threat: the Americanization of our treasured medicare. Canadians may not be enamoured of cuts to health care, the thinking went, but they absolutely hate the thought of American-style health care. The American system, as we have been told again and again, is more expensive than ours yet inaccessible to millions of people. Electing Reformers to the House of Commons could well lead medicare to the same disaster. The Liberals played the "America card." In the dying days of the campaign, both Health Minister David Dingwall and Prime Minister Jean Chrétien made trips west. Both stuck to the message that only Liberals can be trusted with health care.

The success of the strategy was limited but tangible — the Liberals raised enough doubts about their opponents to win a handful of seats in the city centres of Edmonton and Vancouver despite the Reform tide that swept the west. The seats clinched for the party a razor-thin majority government. In short, the America card had saved the Liberals.

Fearmongering about American health care has been a common

theme in political campaigns, both federal and provincial, for many years. In the 1988 federal campaign, for example, the debate about the Free Trade Agreement was coloured by the possible implications to medicare.

But our obsession with American comparisons isn't limited to political campaigns. Such comparisons occur in practically any discussion of medicare. The politician on an open-line radio program is quick to mention "American health care costs" when responding to a caller's angry question on waiting lists. When writing about two-tiered health care in a newspaper column, the political pundit points out that there are millions of uninsured Americans. The policy analyst notes at a public forum that polls consistently show that an overwhelming majority of Canadians prefer the medicare system to an American-style one.

The extent to which the American health care system dominates discussions about medicare is surprising. Why don't Canadians ever refer to, say, Britain's National Health Service (NHS)? Like the medicare system, NHS is a publicly administered program that covers all medical services. The British have run into similar problems (e.g., waiting lists and limited technology). Indeed, the British experimentation with state-run health care led Canadian politicians in part to openly contemplate the idea in Canada. Or what about the German system? Again, the similarities between the two systems are striking, but only the most obscure and technical literature draws comparisons.

Instead, Canadians remain fixated on their American neighbours. The debate about medicare has become dominated by perceptions of so-called private medicine in the United States. For this reason, it is worth exploring the America card, for without a true understanding of the real problem with American health care, it is impossible to identify the source of our medicare woes.

3.2 The America Card

Perhaps part of the strength of the America card is the anti-Americanism it evokes. True, Americans are our largest trading partner, and their culture has many profound influences on Canadians — we watch their movies and TV shows, we read their novels and magazines, we patronize their restaurant and fast-food chains. And, at the end of the day, there's no country Canada is more alike than the United States. But Canadians hate being confused with Americans. After all, we like to think of ourselves as being distinct from our American neighbours. Canada has an envy, bordering on hatred, of the United States — sibling rivalry on a national scale.

Health care is an area where Canada is different from the United States. Universal health care coverage doesn't exist south of the border. Medicare is supposedly a very Canadian way (and a very un-American way) of dealing with health care delivery: it is collective in nature.

Arguments in favour of medicare thus encompass a strong anti-Americanism that appeals to Canadians. Pollster Angus Reid captures this sentiment well in his nostalgic *Shakedown: How the New Economy Is Changing Our Lives*: "Far more persuasive in making the point that we really were a different society was the national medicare system intro-duced by the federal Liberals during the 1960s, borrowed from the Saskatchewan NDP. Medicare was like a badge that said that Canadians did things differently than Americans did — notably, with more com-passion" (281).

There is, of course, more to the America card than simple anti-Americanism. When Minister of Health David Dingwall addressed the Canadian Medical Association's annual meeting in August 1996, he faced a difficult task. Conference delegates were about to vote on a se-ries of motions that would in effect endorse major changes to medi-care, including two-tiered health care. Dingwall wanted to discourage them, yet he knew that many of their concerns were legitimate. He decided to play the America card — about a quarter of his speech re-volved around bashing US health care and the argument that changes to medicare may well open the door to the American health disaster. He told the physicians and surgeons in attendance that medicare does have its problems, but he urged them to look at the American system, in which there are higher overall expenditures, 40 million uninsured citizens, and relatively high administrative costs. He therefore con-cluded that a single-tiered system is the best possible. Any corruption of it, such as allowing people to pay more to get additional services, would be a mistake. "Those who could not afford the insurance would not have access. . . . That's two-tiered medicine. It's not on."

The substance of his speech had been repeated many times before and has been repeated many times since. Politicians often talk about the Americanization of Canadian health care when they oppose reform measures. The America card is a winning political move — deal it suc-cessfully to your opponents and they are sunk. In the fall of 1993, for example, the Manitoba government called five by-elections. The governing Progressive Conservatives were riding high in the polls and hoped to do well in the midterm vote. Political staffers quietly speculated that the party could win two or even three of the seats. The opposition New Democrats focused on one issue: health care. Their message was simple: vote NDP if you want to prevent the Americanization of medicare. The strategy worked like a charm. The Tory vote collapsed, and the ruling party lost all five by-elections. The loss was due almost entirely to the fact that the Conservative government had introduced a series of reform efforts, including the hiring of an American health care consultant to identify waste and redundancy within Manitoba's largest hospital. The Filmon government learned from its mistake. Two years later, Premier Gary Filmon was reelected with a majority government — after he had replaced the minister of health, slowed all major health initiatives, and increased health funding significantly.

In Alberta, a big challenge to Premier Ralph Klein's reelection bid in 1997 occurred in his own political backyard. A physician and longtime Tory fought for the party's nomination in Klein's constituency, charging that the government's health care reforms were leading to an Americanization of the system. Although Klein easily won the party's nod, the embarrassment sparked strong action. Recognizing the potential for his opponents to play the America card, he promptly apologized for his health care reforms, pledged his support to the Canada Health Act, and vowed to pump more money into the system. He then handily won reelection.

Smart political strategies usually capitalize on people's beliefs and fears. The strength of the America card is no exception. Canadians believe that the American system of health care is not only inferior to ours but also completely undesirable. Additionally, Canadians fear that elements of the American system might be found one day within our beloved medicare. This is why Dingwall spent so much time talking about the American system when he addressed the CMA.

3.3 Canadian Perceptions

It has been said that Americans have a benevolent ignorance of Canada, whereas Canadians have a malevolent knowledge of the United States. When it comes to health care, this statement is certainly true. Canadians are well aware that Americans complain often — and with justification — about their health care system.

We see on *ABC News with Peter Jennings* stories about millions of people who are uninsured. We read in our newspapers about the inequity of care in the United States; studies consistently show that the rich get better medical treatment than the poor. We hear on the radio about the incredible costs associated with basic medical treatment south of the border, yet corporations are making billions of dollars. For many Canadians, American health care seems to represent the worst possible system — it's expensive, unreliable, and elitist.

In an interview on 29 May 1997, health economist Cynthia Ramsay summarized the Canadian view with the comment that, "For many Canadians, Americanization evokes images of selling health care on street corners to the highest bidder while millions of uninsured Americans are left to die in the streets." Bearing this in mind, it isn't entirely surprising that polls show Canadians overwhelmingly prefer their system over the American one. A Harris poll in 1988 found that, given a choice, 95% of Canadians would keep their model; only two percent preferred the American model.

3.4 American Admiration

While we have little love for the American approach to health care, some Americans seem to like what we do in Canada.

Senator Edward Kennedy's comments on medicare are flattering. At a Montreal hospital fundraiser in 1996, he said, "Your accomplishment [of universal access] is the envy of every US citizen who understands what you have done" (qtd. in Heinrich). Over the years, Kennedy has heaped praise on the Canadian system in interviews, speeches, and Senate debates. He even appeared on a popular television show, *Chicago Hope*, to tout the advantages of our health care system. And he's not the only prominent American politician to praise medicare. At the height of her influence, First Lady Hillary Clinton declared that the United States should borrow the best aspects of the Canadian system, and she proposed a new model for American health care that would have dramatically expanded the government's role in the sector.

Some Democratic legislators thought that Clinton-care (the reform initiatives proposed by the White House in the fall of 1993) didn't go far enough. Led by Jim McDermott, they called for a Canadian-style plan:

Although universal coverage and other basic principles of President Clinton's health care plan have been widely applauded on Capitol Hill, a brigade of congressional Democrats is fighting for a dark-horse alternative: a government financed system modeled after Canada's. It [the proposal] is already backed by a third of the House's Democratic majority. . . . (Houston)

In the end, McDermott's American Health Security Act didn't get very far. But the large number of Democrats who signed on — 83 congressional representatives from across the country — is impressive given that neither Speaker Tom Foley nor President Bill Clinton were on-side. And dozens of groups openly supported the measure, including Consumers Union, Public Citizen, the National Association of Social Workers, and the American Federation of State, County and Municipal Employees (Houston). McDermott hasn't been the only Democratic Congressman to contemplate a single-tiered system. In 1992, Congressman Marty Russo publicly advocated Canadian-style health care. The topic has been debated on and off for decades.

A typical example of this favourable American view of medicare can be seen in the work of Families USA Foundation, a liberal lobby group based in Washington. Shortly after Clinton's election in 1992 (on a platform of introducing universal health care), the organization published *Looking North for Health: What We Can Learn from Canada's Health Care System*. The analysis in the book is weak, and the basic problems with medicare are glossed over (waiting lists are mentioned only once — and in a positive light), but it does say much about American perceptions of the Canadian health care system. A prominent and respected senator opens the book with a glowing review of the Canadian system, and one of the chapter titles is "Understanding the Health Care System That Works." In the last chapter, Ron Pollack, the executive director of Families USA Foundation, endorses the concept of single-tiered health care. That an influential consumer group would throw its support behind the Canadian system to such an extent speaks volumes about American perceptions of medicare.

Over the years, medicare has been portrayed in a favourable light in articles, editorials, and letters to the editor in publications such as the *Chicago Tribune*, the *New York Times*, *Newsweek*, *Time*, and the *New England Journal of Medicine*. Even corporate executives have publicly flirted with the idea of public insurance. The media reported that Lee

Iacocca, formerly the CEO of Chrysler, gazed "longingly northward to a Canadian system which is seen as a panacea" (Goodman).

Many Americans do see medicare as a superior way of dealing with the issues that both countries confront. Nonetheless, most American politicians have never supported the adoption of a medicare-style system in the United States. And most Americans probably don't understand the Canadian system at all. Their love for it is probably based partly on general misunderstanding and partly on benevolent ignorance. Nevertheless, their curiosity — the respectful interest of a much-envied older sibling — has helped to reaffirm Canadians' belief in medicare.

3.5 Beyond the Myths

Our large neighbour does have troubles with its health care system. But its problems are very different from what Canadians perceive them to be.

What lessons can Canadians learn from the problems of the American system? To answer this question, we need to explore the American health care system in some detail, for much of what Canadians believe about it simply isn't true.

The following five beliefs are especially prevalent, and we'll look at each of them in detail.

1. American health care costs substantially more than Canadian health care.
2. Historically, medicare has been much better at controlling the rise in health expenditures than the free-market alternative in the United States.
3. The American health care system is free market.
4. Uninsured Americans are the poorest in society and represent the government's failure to get involved in health care.
5. The high administrative expenses inherent in an American-style system are wasteful and inefficient.

Not one of the five statements is really true — each one is a myth. This status doesn't prevent our politicians from repeating them time and again as facts. In Dingwall's CMA address, for example, four of the five points were either mentioned or implied. Let's examine each myth.

MYTH 1

American health care costs substantially more than Canadian health care.

> Today we spend over 9% of GDP on health care. The United States spends close to 14%. . . . [Looking at this and other comparisons,] the point is a single-payer publicly funded system is inherently superior.
> — David Dingwall, address to the 129th Annual Meeting
> of the Canadian Medical Association, 19 August 1996

Defenders of medicare like to emphasize that Americans pay more for their health care. As in the above quotation, this argument is usually based on a comparison of expenditures expressed as a percentage of the GDP. In other words, the portion of money spent on health care is compared to the overall wealth of the nation. The higher the percentage, then, the more the system costs. International comparisons are often done in such a way.

There's no question that Americans spend more on health care, but a direct comparison with how much Canadians spend isn't enough. Gross indicators, such as total health expenditures, are a crude instrument for comparison because they don't take into account differences between countries. In fact, the gap in health expenditures (about four percent) is smaller than it seems for several reasons.

A. *Demographics:* The population of the United States is slightly older than Canada's, resulting in higher costs associated with the greater medical needs of an older population.

B. *Legal systems:* American civil trials are often decided by juries (as opposed to judges in Canada) with a long history of awarding damages to plaintiffs to punish defendants. The legal difference has resulted in a malpractice craze in the United States, pushing up malpractice insurance premiums for physicians and thus resulting in higher overall costs.

C. *Research and development:* R & D spending is much higher in the United States, and it inflates the percentage of GDP expenditures, but Canada directly benefits from the technological and pharmaceutical innovations.

D. *Capital spending:* Canadian calculations don't include capital spending (e.g., hospital building and renovating) to the same extent that the US numbers do.

E. *Cross-border care:* Many Canadians go south for their medical care. Because crude comparisons don't take this fact into account, American figures are inflated and Canadian stats are lowered.

F. *Social differences:* Health care consumption in the United States is higher than that in Canada partly because of different social conditions. There are proportionately many more cases of AIDS, spinal injury due to assault, and children suffering from fetal drug exposure.

On the surface, these factors may seem inconsequential. Is a difference in health research significant enough to merit consideration? Yes. Canadians spend little on R & D compared with their American counterparts — Canada's entire research budget is smaller than the R & D budget of the University of Texas–M.D. Anderson Cancer Center (Abraham).

Two Canadian health care consultants, Jacques Krasny and Ian Ferrier, attempted to calculate the effects of such factors on health care expenditures in the respected international journal *Health Affairs*. Using various statistics, they estimated how much the Canadian expenditure percentage would have to be adjusted to create a "fair comparison" (152). They focused their efforts on three areas: health benefits, population mix, and research and development. Using 1991 statistics, for instance, they observed that,

> In the United States, the cohort age sixty-five and over is 1.2 percent larger than in Canada (as a percentage of population), with a resulting net impact on U.S. health care costs of 5.3%. That is, if the Canadian system were required to look after a population with the same demographic profile as in the United States, it would face a 5.3 percent increase in its health care costs. (153)

For this reason, they raised the Canadian GDP figure by 0.5%.

After many similarly reasoned calculations, Krasny and Ferrier estimated that the gap in spending as a fraction of GDP is less than a quarter of the number that is so widely reported. And they noted that many of the differences can't be measured, differences such as the large number of Vietnam vets in the United States, malpractice liability and insurance, intense American urbanization, and hidden administrative costs in Canada. They concluded that, "Given the intensely conservative nature of our adjustment components, more sophisticated analysis would likely yield the result that the Canadian system costs as much as, or slightly more than the US system" (154).

Krasny and Ferrier aren't alone in this view. In a recent article in the *Wall Street Journal*, Dr. Jerome C. Arnett Jr. makes a similar point: "If Canada had comparable social problems with drugs and the like, its per capita spending on health care would surely be greater than that of the US." Such analysis isn't without its critics. Daniel R. Waldo and Sally T. Sonnefeld have suggested that Krasny and Ferrier are off base. They disagree with the extent to which Krasny and Ferrier adjust for factors such as capital costs.[1] Interestingly, while they argue that Krasny and Ferrier have somewhat overcompensated in their calculations, they also believe that adjustments should be made for a fair comparison. They conclude that the "correct" difference in spending is about 20% lower than the unadjusted figure (161).

The "real" difference between spending in the two countries is practically impossible to determine. It's safe to assume that this difference probably lies somewhere between the two estimates. But whether you accept the Waldo-Sonnefeld figure or the Krasny-Ferrier adjustment, straight comparisons between the health expenditures are clearly misleading.

But let's not get carried away with technical arguments about capital costs and the like — the exact difference between health care spending in the two countries isn't that important. What is significant is that practically no analysis has been done in Canada on the unadjusted figures despite the frequency of the crude comparison. The most popular book on medicare, *Strong Medicine*, makes much of the difference in spending but doesn't mention that the comparison is flawed (see Rachlis and Kushner 188–218).

Even taking into account these factors, Americans still spend more of their GDP on health. But what does this fact really mean? Health care experts and politicians tout it as though it's proof that one system is superior to the other. It isn't.

International comparisons (e.g., by the United Nations) often measure quality of life and affluence by how high a fraction of income a country spends on housing, recreation, and travel. Why is it that money spent on these things is good yet high health expenditures are not? Or consider education. A common Canadian (and United Nations) criticism of the United States is that not enough of its GDP is spent on education. Why do our politicians argue that Canada has a better public school system than that in the United States because we invest more money in education and that Canada has a superior health care system because we spend less on it?

International comparisons in this regard rarely make sense. They amount to a "Lada Argument": the Lada is the best car in the world because it's the cheapest. Sure, a Volvo may be safer, a Camry more comfortable, and a Probe faster. But the Lada is the cheapest — and that's what matters.

The Lada Argument is ridiculous; strangely, though, when experts discuss health care, it is widely accepted. Quality cannot be measured by expenditures as a percentage of GDP. If Dingwall really believed his own argument, he would have added that Turkey has an even better health care system — that country spends well under five percent of its GDP on health.

Some economists have even forwarded the argument that Canada is worse off for the lower spending. In "A Thriving Health Care Sector Could Contribute to a Health Economy," Cynthia Ramsay and Michael Walker argue that part of the reason for higher unemployment in Canada as opposed to the United States is lower health care spending. Based on an analysis from the *Financial Post*, they conclude that Canada loses about 100,000 jobs a year to the United States in health care (21).

Here's the real question: do Canadians have an efficient and effective health care system? That is, given the amount of money we spend on health care, do our citizens receive quality care? A simple numerical statistic such as 9.5% fails to answer these questions (though it does make for solid political rhetoric).

It's interesting to note how often advocates of medicare draw on such a meaningless barrage of statistics and facts to "prove" that Canada has a better health care system than that of the United States. For instance, how often should people visit their doctors? In the United States, people see, on average, a physician 5.5 times a year. In Canada, the number of physician contacts is 6.9. But what does this higher rate mean? Such statistics can be spun out effortlessly — the same stat can be used to argue that Canadians have better access to physicians or that Americans have a more efficient system that requires fewer visits to doctors.

Such crude statistics tell us practically nothing. After all, the relevant information is not how many times we and our southern neighbours sit in physicians' waiting rooms a year but the quality of those visits. How quickly can we see physicians when we need to? How qualified and skilled are these doctors? What tests are available to help a diagnosis?

In *Universal Health Care: What the United States Can Learn from the Canadian Experience*, the Armstrongs can't answer any of these questions, but they get around the problem of crude statistics with a simplistic solution — wherever these comparisons differ, the Americans are in the wrong. Canada has more hospital beds per capita. Excellence! The United States has more hospital workers per bed. Waste! Canada has more nurses and more highly trained nurses. Efficiency! The United States has more doctors and more highly trained specialists. Redundancy! Canadians stay in hospitals longer, have more nursing homes, and undergo more lung transplants — all illustrative of the strength of our compassionate public system. Americans have more diagnostic equipment, higher administrative costs, and more heart bypass surgeries — all illustrative of the deficiency of a greedy, for-profit system.

Expenditures as a percentage of GDP, hospital beds per capita, and so on — such statistics are of limited value.

MYTH 2

Historically, medicare has been much better at controlling the rise in health expenditures than the free-market alternative in the United States.

> For the pre-medicare period, health spending grew from the same level and at the same rate in both countries as a share of GNP. In both, the share increased from 5% to over 7%. In the nearly twenty-five years of Canadian medicare, the growth rate has sharply diverged. . . . The doubling of the GNP share in the US compares to a much more modest growth in Canada from 7% to about 10% in the same period. . . . Canada's system has achieved a greater containment of costs.
>
> — Michael Decter, *Healing Medicare* (210)

Canadian experts often speak of the two countries' growth in health care expenditures. The point is that health care costs in the United States have exploded under its free-market system, whereas Canada's medicare system has helped to control costs because of its great efficiency. This argument was particularly popular in the late 1980s.

On the surface, the numbers appear to support this assertion. Let's look at a 20-year period. In 1967, Canada and the United States spent about the same percentage of GDP on health care — 6.38%. In 1987, Canada spent 8.98% of GDP, whereas the United States spent over 11.06%. The growth rates appear to be unequal.

This argument is deceptive because it fails to take into account what a percentage of GDP really is: a fraction. In other words, the statistic so often used isn't a direct measure of expenditures; rather, it measures health care as a percentage of GDP.[2] Remember that the growth of a fraction can be caused by changes in either the numerator (health care spending) or the denominator (GDP). For example, the percentage of GDP on health expenditures for a country could double if, say, the GDP drops by 50% — the money actually spent on hospitals, doctors, and the like hasn't changed, but the GDP has. And the converse is true: a country could dramatically increase spending in health care but not show a significant change in the percentage of GDP if the GDP itself has grown over the same period.

This latter situation is relevant to "cost containment." Over a 20-year period from 1967 to 1987, Canada's real GDP grew by about 74% per capita, but the GDP of the United States only grew by 38%. In other words, a straight comparison based on spending as a percentage of GDP produces a skewed conclusion. If we look at health care spending alone, rather than as a fraction of GDP, we come to a very different conclusion. In 1967, Canada spent about 75% of what the United States spent per person. And, in 1987, the spending of the two countries was about the same. Over that period, the growth in health care spending per person was almost identical: 4.58% here, 4.38% there.

Now, in fairness to the argument about cost containment, there does appear to be a divergence in growth rates over the past half-decade. Americans are spending more money on a per capita basis than Canadians. But when medicare was a popular program — that is, during the first two decades, when waiting lists were minimal, new technologies were generally accessible, and physicians took pride in the service — the growth rates in the two countries were in fact identical. Historically, the Canadian system has been no better at cost control than the American system.

But for all the rhetoric about cost containment, it isn't clear what the consequences of this goal are. In a system in which most of the money spent is budgeted by the government (at both the provincial and the federal levels), cost containment can be achieved by the government simply not allocating money.

Again, the use of crude international comparisons fails to address the real issue: is medicare providing Canadians with an efficient and effective health care system?

MYTH 3

The American health care system is free market.

> The proposition that government get out of health care altogether can only imply a market-driven, corporately-based health care system.
> That is exactly what exists in the United States.
>
> — Dr. Michael Gordon,
> letter to the *Medical Post*, 3 June 1997

Canadians have long assumed that comparisons between the health care systems in Canada and the United States illustrate the direct contrast between a public system and a private system. We happily speak about our "free" health care and express concern about the fact that Americans must pay for their care.

But this rhetoric is simplistic: health care, after all, is more than a patient seeing his family physician. Proper medical care involves many different professionals, including nurses, dentists, optometrists, chiropractors, technicians, and pharmacists. Health care also encompasses diagnostic tests, pharmaceutical drugs, and hospital care. Many of the health services in Canada aren't covered by medicare. Dental care falls into this category. When you see the dentist, you pay out of pocket or, more likely, your insurance company will pay for the expenses above a certain level.

Because coverage varies from province to province, other services (e.g., chiropractic care) may be publicly financed in one province but not in another. And some services are only partially covered. Pharmaceutical drugs, for example, are free to needy citizens.

Many services are completely covered by the public system. They are termed "medically necessary," though the term is loosely applied and often involves procedures that aren't life saving. This last category includes hospital stays, checkups with a family physician, and a whole gambit of diagnostic tests.

According to the Organization for Economic Cooperation and Development Health Data, when it's all put together, the government pays for approximately 70% of all medical expenditures in Canada. Clearly, most of the expenses are picked up by the state — but certainly not all of them.

And while there's no question that the American health care system is different from the Canadian one, government funding of health care in the United States is far from minimal. In fact, according to the National

Center for Policy Analysis, the federal, state, and local levels of government directly pay for about 46% of all medical care (W17). For every dollar spent by the private sector, about one dollar is spent by the government. The bulk of this public spending goes to two big programs: Medicare and Medicaid. Medicare covers the medical expenses of Americans over the age of 65, and Medicaid provides for the care of the poorest citizens.

Direct public spending on health care in the United States, then, is significant. The government also offers tax subsidies for health care. Factoring them into the equation, we find that 56% of all health care spending in the United States comes from the public purse (National Center for Policy Analysis).

The various levels of government do more than simply spend money — they also tend to regulate health care. Many laws have been passed that influence how insurance companies conduct themselves — from expensive procedures that they must cover to limitations on cost containment. Both federal and state legislators have drafted tens of thousands of pages of regulations in recent years. And the trend toward greater regulation has hardly waned since the Republican sweep of Congress. In 1995, for example, Congress mandated insurance companies to cover mental disorders, just like other ailments, and to cover the first 48 hours in hospital for new mothers. In 1997, Republican flirtations with federal health regulations included coverage of contraceptives (Senator Olympia Snowe), new restrictions on Health Maintenance Organizations (HMOs) and other types of health care insurance (Senator Alfonse D'Amato), and coverage of uninsured children (Senator Orin Hatch) (Rees). With an off-year election, 1998 saw Republicans push a new batch of regulations under the auspices of a Patients' Bill of Rights, including the right of a woman to see a gynecologist without referral and the right of patients not to be refused ER care. If a generally antiregulatory group of Republicans is pushing for such measures, there's no question that the influence of government in health care delivery in the United States is growing.

The *New York Times* reports that many of the regulations contemplated by Congress have already been adopted by state legislatures. Regulations have included allowing patients to visit doctors outside their HMO network for an additional charge (16 states), outlawing restrictions on doctor-patient communication (46 states), assuring that women can directly see a gynecologist/obstetrician without a referral from another doctor or allowing women to designate such specialists as their primary care providers (36 states), and requiring that HMOs cover all emergency services when a "prudent lay person" would consider them necessary (23 states) (Pear).

In short, the American health care system is dominated by government spending and regulations. It can hardly be considered "free market."

MYTH 4

Uninsured Americans are the poorest in society and represent the government's failure to get involved in health care.

> We must never forget we spend about 9% of GDP to produce a first-rate system that provides access to all Canadians. Americans spend 13% of GDP on a system that leaves 30 million [sic] without coverage. That, to me, speaks to a wonderful marriage of compassion and efficiency.
> — Angus Reid, *Shakedown* (341)

The high number of uninsured citizens is an aspect of the American health care system that Canadians find profoundly disturbing. The uninsured, we assume, are the poorest of citizens. A lack of insurance is equated with an inability to receive medical care. Consider, for example, the comment made by Diane Francis in a column for the *Financial Post*: "There are now 43 million Americans without health care" ("Random Facts"). An interesting mistake — there are 43 million Americans without *health insurance*. For many Canadians — including those who, like Francis, are enormously critical of the medicare system — the uninsured are assumed to have no health care.

With this frame of mind, the American health care system seems not only undesirable but also cruel. *How can Americans do that to the poor?* we ask ourselves with seemingly justified moral disgust. Health care, after all, is a basic need. *Can you imagine four million people in Canada without, say, proper shelter or clothing?*

In this light, low-income America begins to look less like low-income Canada and more like a scene reminiscent of the ghetto in Victor Hugo's *Les Misérables*. Such an image, however, runs counter to the results of the 1993 survey of uninsured Americans by Novalis Corporation. Half of the uninsured — those Americans presumably without any health care whatsoever — rated their medical care as "good" or "excellent" (Frum, *What's Right* 104). Amazingly, that level of satisfaction is about the same as that of the elderly covered by Medicare.

The uninsured, it turns out, aren't the poorest of citizens. The black, unemployed, single mother with three young children living in south-central Los Angeles — whom we assume to have been forgotten by the callous free-market system — isn't one of the uninsured masses. She's on Medicaid. Her children are on Medicaid. And probably her neighbours are on Medicaid.

Nor are the uninsured deprived of medical care. Although they tend to utilize physicians' services less frequently than insured Americans, they aren't strangers to doctors' offices. In a *Wall Street Journal* poll, 81% saw a physician within the previous three years. Among the insured, the percentage was only slightly higher at 87% ("American Opinion").

Economists John Goodman and Gerald Musgrave provided a detailed analysis of the situation in *Patient Power: Solving America's Health Care Crisis*. On the topic of the uninsured, they note that

> It is believed widely in this country, and even more prevalently in Europe, that uninsured residents in the United States are routinely denied health care. That belief is quite wrong. What is true is that the existence or non-existence of health insurance makes a big difference in determining how care is paid for. (355)

Who, then, are the uninsured? Forget *Les Misérables*. Imagine, instead, a college campus. The uninsured tend to be young Americans — 60% are under the age of 35. Many are out of high school or university, beginning their first jobs. Even more surprising is that they tend not to stay uninsured for very long. Over a 28-month period, only 4.8% had no insurance for the entire time (Goodman and Musgrave 356).[3] On any given day, only about half of the uninsured were without coverage. The pool of people we define as uninsured is constantly changing as some people gain insurance and others lose it. Although the concept of lacking insurance may seem foreign to Canadians, the situation isn't unlike unemployment. At various points in their lives, many people will be without jobs. Unemployment, however, is temporary for the vast majority. Only a small percentage of the overall population is unemployed. And, of these people, only a small percentage remains unemployed indefinitely. And, as with the unemployed, most people consider the high number of uninsured Americans undesirable.

Uninsured Americans have opted for a "pay-as-you-go" approach to health care. But why would they choose not to buy insurance? One of the most basic problems with American health care is the extent to which the government has set out regulations and rules. Insurance companies are expected to cover a dizzying array of procedures from the life saving to the purely cosmetic: "heart transplants in Georgia, liver transplants in Illinois, hairpieces in Minnesota, marriage counseling in California, and deposits to sperm banks in Massachusetts" (Goodman and Musgrave 47).

The numerous regulations partly reflect the politicization of health care in the United States. Because so many special interests have discovered the enormous payoffs of state regulations, they spend millions every year lobbying to have the required coverage extended.

Make no mistake — many of the required regulations allow people to get very expensive services at reasonable costs. For a couple seeking marriage counselling in California or for a bald man in Minnesota, mandated coverage is fantastic. But the more services that must be covered, the higher the premiums must ultimately become. After all, the money for hairpieces and counselling has to come from somewhere — and insurance companies are like any other business: the costs borne by them get passed on to the consumer. Imagine the cost of a car if the government required every manufacturer to include automatic transmission, power windows, air conditioning, and antilock brakes.

The situation with medical health insurance in the United States isn't that different. As a result, people with lower-income jobs find that even the most basic insurance comes with high premiums. A simple insurance policy for a medical catastrophe doesn't exist — it must include a state-required sea of services. Consider that 45 states require health insurance coverage for the services of chiropractors, four states mandate coverage for acupuncture, and two states require coverage for naturopaths (who specialize in prescribing herbs). At least 13 states limit the ability of insurers to avoid covering people who have AIDS or are at a high risk of getting AIDS. Forty states mandate coverage for alcoholism, 27 states mandate coverage for drug addiction, and 29 states mandate coverage for mental illness. Seven states even mandate coverage for in vitro fertilization (Goodman and Musgrave 47).

The explosion in mandated coverage — from eight such regulations in 1960 to just under 1,000 in 1991 — pushes up the cost of insurance. Two professors actually calculated the increases to premiums caused by certain mandated coverage: 6–8% for substance abuse, 10–13% for outpatient mental health care, and up to 21% for psychiatric hospital care for employee dependants (Jensen and Morrisey 48).

In a *Washington Times* article, Grace-Marie Arnett and Melindia Schriver, both of the Galen Institute, outline state regulations in recent years. Between 1990 and 1994, 16 states passed stringent health insurance regulations, many aimed at reducing the number of uninsured citizens in those states. The regulations included such benevolent ideas as requiring an insurer to sell a policy to anyone who applies and agrees to pay the premium, even if that person is already sick; mandating treatment coverage for certain illnesses; and forcing an insurer to charge the same price to anyone in the community, regardless of health status.

The irony is that the regulations ended up having the opposite effect to that intended. By 1996, the uninsured populations in these 16 states had grown an average of eight times faster than in the 34 states with less comprehensive regulations or no regulations. In 1990, the two groups of states had nearly equal rates of growth in coverage. But could this difference have been due to other economic factors? It turns out that the 16 states had employment and income characteristics similar to those of the rest of the nation.

Most working Americans receive their health insurance through their employers' plans. With rising premiums, a growing number of employers are choosing not to provide employees with such health benefits,[4] particularly those in entry-level, low-paying jobs — just the sort of jobs young Americans are likely to get. These citizens must make a choice — they can buy health insurance with their own money (with after-tax dollars), or they can refuse to buy it. Many choose the latter option. The phenomenon of the uninsured is the result. As writer David Frum observed, "America has millions of uninsured people for the same reason that it would have millions of naked people if the only clothing stores permitted to operate were Bendel's and Saks" (*What's Right* 112).

MYTH 5

The high administrative expenses inherent in an American-style system are wasteful and inefficient.

Each province in Canada operates a single, large health insurance plan, and this federal-provincial single-payer system is the main reason our administrative costs are so well controlled. By contrast, there are more than 1,500 "payers" in the United States, which means 1,500 sets of actuaries,

1,500 computer systems, and 1,500 sets of high-paid executives. The cost and complexity are further compounded by the fact that each company offers a multiplicity of plans.

— Michael Rachlis and Carol Kushner, *Strong Medicine* (194)

Many proponents of medicare praise it for administrative efficiency. The argument is straightforward: because of the administrative simplicity of a single-payer system, medicare is a cheaper alternative to the endless paperwork seen in the United States. This argument isn't new. It was one of the original arguments raised for the establishment of medicare in the 1960s. "This primarily single-payer system was adopted not only because it was the most equitable," note medicare advocates Armstrong and Armstrong in *Wasting Away: The Undermining of Canadian Health Care*, "but also because it was the cheapest. It was cheaper mainly because it reduced administrative costs . . ." (156).

There's no question that the American health care system has higher administrative expenses than the Canadian system. The United States spends about .59% of GDP on administrative overhead versus 0.11% in Canada. But is this really proof of the inherent superiority of the Canadian system? For many people, the answer is a resounding yes. The term "administrative expenditures" implies waste because administration is equated with bureaucracy.

This view is simplistic, as Dr. Kenneth E. Thorpe, a professor of health policy and administration, explains in a highly praised paper: "The most critical assumption is that each health plan engages in the same administrative activities and pursues the same goals. Thus the plan with the lowest level of administrative spending is the most efficient, with higher levels representing waste. The basic assumption underlying these comparisons is incorrect, however" (42). Administrative activities amount to more than "paper shuffling." Of course, many of these activities aren't necessary in Canada. They reflect efforts, for example, to gain an edge over the competition. Hence, major insurance companies will spend money on ads in the Sunday *New York Times*, staff a sales division for every region of the country, secure the services of Weiden&Kennedy for advertising expertise, and cosponsor the US Open to raise their profile in the community. These costs can't be avoided in the private sector — but they aren't incurred under a government-run system. The Ontario government, for instance, doesn't need to place a full-page ad in the *Toronto Star* espousing the virtues of medicare and encouraging Torontonians to "take their illnesses" to a public hospital.

We must be careful how far we take this argument. After all, the post office of the 1960s was hardly a bastion of efficiency just because it didn't need to advertise for customers. A legislated monopoly allows employees to set their own paces. Individual expenditures (e.g., marketing) may be higher in a private sector system, but the bigger picture — that is, the total efficiency of the system — is a different matter. Competition, after all, pushes organizations toward efficiency. In a government monopoly, such trends don't exist. In *Public Choice II*, University of Vienna economist Dennis Mueller presents his survey of 50 studies comparing government and private provision of goods and services. In only two cases did government firms perform better.

And there's another side to the administrative coin. Many such activities are legitimate. For example, tracking costs is useful to both health providers and insurance companies alike. A well-developed administrative system can allow health providers to identify areas of waste and duplication — by knowing how funds are spent, they can attempt to find ways of spending the money better. Administration may seem undesirable, but it facilitates billing and clinical data that are beneficial to both medical education and clinical and health services research. Thorpe concludes that "Americans have invested heavily in managed care information and data-processing systems, which add to administrative costs but are widely thought to reduce health care spending. These investments provide both clinical and financial information used for total quality management and research on patient outcomes and quality" (54).

It's ironic that many who tout Canada's low administrative spending as a virtue also recognize that not enough information is available on clinical utilization. But we can't admire the wealth of the businesswoman but resent her thrift, for it's her thrift that has allowed her to retain her wealth. This section, for example, opens with a quotation from *Strong Medicine* that berates the American health care system for administrative overhead; later the authors bemoan the fact that little information is available on clinical utilization (see Rachlis and Kushner 231).

The issue of administrative expenses does, however, raise an interesting question: does the United States spend too much on administration? Sure, a certain amount of spending may reduce overall costs, but don't we see too much of a good thing south of the border? The answer, probably, is yes. For reasons explored below, overhead could be reduced. The problem, however, isn't sufficient to throw out the whole system, as some American politicians have suggested. Nor is it justification for a feeling of Canadian superiority, as some health care experts have forwarded. Rather, it suggests that the American health care system is in need of reform to allow insurance companies to reduce expenses so that premiums can be kept low.

3.6 The Source of the Problem

Between public programs (Medicare, Medicaid, Veterans' Affairs) and private insurance, American patients pay very little directly for their health care expenses. Depending on the insurance coverage, the odds are that a New Yorker with a brain tumour will enjoy top-notch care without ever having to reach for his chequebook. The huge hospital bill, the countless doctors' visits, the MRI scans and blood tests, the neurosurgery — although the expenses may be tens of thousands of dollars, the insurance company will foot the bulk of the bill.

Patients, of course, don't always view things this way. To a single, working mother with limited insurance, a hospital stay may mean that she has to cover the expense of her aspirins, tissues, and other essentials. The bill may come to a seemingly outrageous sum of hundreds of dollars. Many hospitals mark up the prices on basic items in order to raise extra revenue. This markup is irritating — but such a bill still reflects a fraction of the total cost to the system.

Most Americans are covered by some form of health insurance, whether public or private. But unlike insurance coverage for the house or boat — policies that tend to cover only high expenses after catastrophic events — health insurance tends to cover nearly everything.

The buffer between the bill and the patient is real. On average, Americans directly pay only five cents for every dollar they spend in a hospital. Put another way, if a patient stays in Chicago's Rush Hospital for three weeks, she will end up paying for just over a day of that entire stay. And for physicians' services, Americans pay only 19¢ for every dollar spent. They average 24¢ on the dollar for other health services (Goodman and Musgrave vii). Americans get a very good deal for what they actually pay out of pocket.

As a result, citizens have little reason to think twice before using health services. Is the common cold reason enough to see a physician? Obviously not. But since patients aren't financially accountable for their choices, it's not surprising that family physicians' offices would be crowded with patients suffering from trivial illnesses such as the common cold. And if Americans have little reason to hesitate before marching off to a doctor's office, they also have little reason to consider the prices of the services they buy. When Goodman and Musgrave contacted seven Dallas hospitals about the cost of a standard blood count, they got seven different prices, ranging from $11.00 to $33.25 (174). Big-ticket items had similar discrepancies: child birth ranged from $1,069 to $2,024 (175). "The same consumers who would drive across town to save a dollar and a half on a movie ticket neither know nor care what they pay for medical services," notes David Frum, "because the money they save belongs to their employer [or their insurer], not to them" (*What's Right* 106).

The lack of connection between usage and payment results in a virtual spending spree. Consider, for example, the frustration expressed by Dr. Elliot Rosenberg in a letter to the *New York Times*:

> A few days ago the couple came in for a follow-up visit. They were upset. At their daughter's insistence they had gone to an out-of-town neurologist. She wanted the "best" for her father and would spare no (Medicare) expense to get it. The patient had undergone a CT scan, a magnetic resonance imaging, a spinal tap, a brain-stem evoke potential and a carotid duplex ultrasound.
>
> No remediable problems were discovered. The Medicare billing was more than $4000 so far.

Given that the United States has the most advanced high-tech equipment in the world, it's surprising that health care spending isn't higher than it is.

Health care, it turns out, can serve as an incredible sink for money. Dr. John Goodman of the National Center for Policy Analysis calculates that the entire GDP of the United States could be spent on preventive health care if every American was given all of the blood tests currently available (Ferrara, "New Prescription" 27). Put another way, Americans could spend everything they have on health care and then some.

That patients pay so little out of pocket has resulted in two damning trends.

First, administrative expenses have soared. Because insurance policies cover everything from a basic checkup to heart surgery, the amount of paperwork to process all the claims is dizzying. But from an administrative point of view, a $15 claim isn't more difficult to process than a $150 claim. In fact, small claims may cost more to process than the bill they fill.

Second, managed care has proliferated. Because patients have little financial incentive to take responsibility for their actions — as health consumers, they simply take advantage of the situation — those paying for the insurance are forced to try to control costs. In order to fully appreciate this dynamic, we must understand the way in which Americans get their coverage. Carrie J. Gavora, a health policy analyst at the Heritage Foundation, explains that

> Most Americans get their health coverage through their place of work, and the employer selects and owns the plans made available to the employees. This happens because today's tax code gives tax breaks to employees on the value of their health plan, but only if their employer purchases it. This leads to the perverse situation in which employers, not families, are making crucial decisions about the type of health plan and benefits their employees receive. (1–2)

Increasingly, employers are looking to managed care companies in order to control health care costs. HMOs account for coverage of 50% of all privately insured workers — and the number is rising (Gawande). Today 84% of workers are subscribed to some other type of managed care. In the past, employers provided many options to their employees. More and more, though, employers are simply subscribing their employees to one plan. According to a study from consulting company KPMG Peat Marwick, 80% of small and medium-sized companies with employee health coverage offer only one plan, and 47% of large companies offer no choice either (Gawande). As Ron Pollack, the director of Families USA, recently observed, "Most of us get our health coverage from an employer, and our employers increasingly are saying 'here's one plan and it's the only plan and you don't have a choice' so you can't, in effect, vote with your feet and thereby drive quality" (qtd. in Gavora 2).

Many Americans are dissatisfied with this development. According to a poll commissioned by the *Wall Street Journal*, Americans believe that HMOs have had a largely detrimental impact on their health care:

hurting the long-term doctor-patient relationship (54%), affecting a doctor's ability to control treatment decisions (54%), and reducing access to specialists (50%) ("American Opinion" A14). The result isn't surprising — as Gavora notes, "The health plan is accountable to the purchaser (the employer), whose primary interest is cost control, rather than the consumer who wants quality" (2).

In many ways, managed care was inevitable. Patients have little need to think about health care costs, but these costs still exist. Employers, desperate to control the spiralling expenditures on health care benefits, are increasingly looking to HMOs. After all, if patients aren't going to make the hard decisions, then someone has to do it for them.

In part, HMOs have a bad reputation because of negative media depictions.[5] Many companies offer quality care at affordable prices. But this isn't always the case. In order to control costs, HMOs try to restrict patients' access to health care, often by employing statistical analysis. (Dr. Michael DeBakey, a pioneering heart surgeon and director of the DeBakey Heart Center at the Baylor College of Medicine, asks: "We would not allow an unqualified clerk to recommend repairs for our car, so why would we settle for one when it comes to our own health?" [qtd. in "Rx"].) They also restrict a doctor's ability to practise medicine as he or she sees fit. The doctor-patient relationship — the building block of health care — is thus compromised.

The irony is that, from an economic perspective, the forces driving change in the United States are remarkably similar to those at work in Canada. American patients don't pay for the bulk of their health expenses. Neither do Canadian patients. Thus, in both countries, health care has evolved into a Sunday brunch at which consumers can feast on expensive items without concern for the cost. They have no incentive to economize.

In the United States, the lack of individual incentive has resulted in a proliferation of managed care. Simply put, patients aren't making the necessary decisions, so insurance companies are doing so on their behalf. In Canada, provincial governments have sought to ration health care through waiting lists. Canadians don't need to fight HMO bureaucrats to get an MRI scan. But they must wait months to get the test because government bureaucrats have limited the availability of scanners.

Government actions have only served to worsen the situation. In Canada, the federal government took a hard line in 1984 and passed the Canada Health Act. It not only prevents any experimentation at the provincial level but also hopelessly limits the role of the private sector and thus competition. In the United States, state legislators have worked hard to regulate the insurance companies by requiring them to cover expensive procedures. Faced with the costs of covering hairpieces (Minnesota), pastoral counselling (Vermont), and sperm bank deposits (Massachusetts), premiums for even the simplest medical insurances for catastrophes have risen and therefore forced more young Americans into the ranks of the uninsured.

3.7 Learning the Real Lesson from the American System

It turns out, then, that the perceptions Canadians have of the American health care system are simply not accurate. Consider again the beliefs stated at the start of this chapter: that the American system is largely private, with little government involvement; that the poor are often uninsured and without proper care; that the administrative costs are high and unavoidable. Why are these beliefs so widely held by Canadians yet so universally untrue?

The irony, of course, is that the two systems are evolving in a similar direction — away from individual decision making and toward bureaucratically managed health care. Not surprisingly, some of medicare's critics have made the point. Dr. Michael Walker, executive director of the Fraser Institute, argued at a panel discussion that health care in the 10 provinces is just like 10 government-run HMOs. He noted wryly that, at least in the United States, the HMOs face competition with one another, while the provincial government plans are legislated monopolies.[6] Walker isn't alone in this analysis. When asked his opinion on the American system, Dr. Jack Armstrong, the soft-spoken former CMA president from Winnipeg, observed, "many believe that we are already in one big HMO."

No doubt Canadians and Americans have very different health care systems, and the point of this chapter isn't to argue that the two systems are identical. Asked about Canadian and American health care, a Canadian doctor practising in the United States responded that the two systems are fundamentally different. His reasons were that (1) state-of-the-art equipment is abundant in the United States; (2) the small fees imposed on American patients increase their personal responsibility; (3) frequent legal action in the United States increases provider accountability; (4) HMOs still compete with each other to be selected by em-

ployers; and (5) in some companies, employees are able to select between several plans, further increasing competition. "Saying that they
[the two systems] are fundamentally similar would be like arguing that
in 1960 American agriculture was the same as Soviet agriculture since
they were both regulated."

The two systems are not fundamentally the same. The economic
problem they suffer from and the resulting trend away from individual
choice, however, are fundamentally similar.

And we could add a sixth difference to the physician's list: many
Americans recognize that the trend toward bureaucratically managed
health care is undesirable. Some insurance companies are experiment-
ing with different models of health care delivery that attempt to match
the needs of the consumers with the financial realities of the companies. As a result, various types of Medical Savings Accounts (MSAs) are
being tried by the major insurance companies with surprising success.
MSAs hold much promise — by empowering patients to make their
own health care decisions, individual choice is restored while needless
administrative expenses are minimized.

But if the two health care systems suffer from a similar economic
problem, why is the American system so vilified in Canada? Clearly,
there are problems with the American system, but nothing comparable
to the myths that are so widely believed.

In *Strong Medicine*, probably the most successful book written on the
Canadian medicare system, Rachlis and Kushner spend an entire chapter attacking the American health care system. The chapter's title, "Lies
about Canada, Myths about America," gives a good indication of their
bias. Typical of their analysis is the discussion of access to high technology. In it, they mention a 1993 article from the *New England Journal
of Medicine* in which Dr. Beverly Morgan observes that patients with
private insurance can get MRI scans in Orange County immediately.
Patients of Medi-Cal, the state-run program for low-income Califor-
nians, are subjected to paperwork and a wait of two to three weeks.

There thus seems to be a problem with Medi-Cal — clearly, clinics
are less eager to deal with the government insurance. To the unbiased
observer, the solution lies in either reducing the paperwork involved in
processing a Medi-Cal claim or increasing payments to health care providers. But to Rachlis and Kushner, the situation indicates the cruel,
elitist nature of American health care: "Dr. Morgan's little experiment
shows, however, that even if MRI scanners were as numerous as

McDonald's outlets, those with no or inadequate access insurance . . . would still face big obstacles to getting a scan when they need one" (*Strong Medicine* 203). The message is clear: Americans may have more high-tech equipment, but Canadians shouldn't be envious, because many Americans can't get access to it. The irony is that the incredible wait Medi-Cal patients must endure — two to three weeks — would be exceptionally short by Canadian standards.

American bashing is a common theme in Canadian analysis. Consider Canada's most popular books on the subject:

- *Strong Medicine*, 346 pages in total, devotes 52 pages to Canada–US comparisons;
- *Universal Health Care* devotes all of its 176 pages to such comparisons;
- *Wasting Away*, 227 pages in length, offers such comparisons on 13 pages; and
- *Healing Health Care* devotes 11 of 256 pages to Canada–US comparisons.

There's practically no sound analysis of the true difference between the two health care systems. Part of this lack is easily explained: politicians (particularly, though certainly not exclusively, of the left) have found the issue to be politically useful. They opportunistically exploit the fears of Canadians. It would be naïve to assume that this is the only instance of opportunism. Other political issues, such as the Free Trade Agreement, have been similarly abused. Political parties hoping to succeed on the campaign trail are thus tempted to play the America card. Not surprisingly, some do.

Other politicians have come to fear this card. They may know the real facts behind the bunk arguments about Americanization, but they remain silent. Politicians in right-wing parties probably realize how pathetic comparisons to the American health care system really are, but they must be careful about the controversy. Why fight a hopeless battle against the America card when there are so many other issues worth taking on that could yield real success? So they choose not to use political capital, and the perceptions continue.

But there's a more disturbing element to these misconceptions. Sure, politicians have exploited the issue, but what about all the experts who should know better? For the most part, health care experts (university professors, Ministry of Health staff, and other health policy analysts) have been the most vocal in touting the superiority of the medicare system. In fact, much of the analysis of medicare has focused on trying to "prove" its superiority over the American alternative. At this point, medicare ceases to be a matter of public policy discussion and instead takes on the characteristics of a cult. Loyal followers defend this cult with an array of rational and irrational arguments. The American system is perceived not only as inferior but also as deviant.

With such a frame of mind, health care experts have adopted a tone of criticism that is not only cutting and offensive but also nearly hysterical. University of British Columbia professors Morris Barer and Robert Evans state in an international journal that those who believe in a private sector-based health care system are captured by special interests or are callously unethical. Michael Decter, former deputy minister of health in Ontario, writes that Canadians shouldn't even think about "dangerous ideas" such as user fees (a modest reform effort that has been adopted in practically every other country with a public health care system) because they will inevitably lead to an American-style system that will destroy quality health care in Canada, for "Adam Smith's invisible hand works less well when wearing a surgical glove. It is neither invisible nor efficient" (20). Rachlis and Kushner go even further: the United States, they suggest, is in a bitter "war" over a Canadian-style system, with greedy insurance companies and the American Medical Association on one side of the battlefield and the needs of millions of Americans on the other. They insist that Canadians get involved: it's not enough for us to be true believers in the Cult of Medicare — we must convert others.

By vilifying the American health care system, Canadian experts have done us a grave disservice. As the United States struggles to deal with problems such as an aging population and escalating health care costs, we can watch and learn from its struggle. Reform efforts in Oregon, Arkansas, and New York may be useful in Ontario, Alberta, and Nova Scotia.

If we can move past the fearmongering and the myths, we can ask a relatively simple question: what can we learn from the American health care system? Canadian experts have long answered this question with a rant about for-profit health care. In fact, the lesson we should learn is more profound: bureaucratic decision making (by either government or HMO officials) is no substitute for individual choice.

4

The Fundamental Flaw

CASE STUDY 1

A middle-aged man feels tightness in his chest after a squash game. The pain worsens and radiates to his left arm. He is rushed to a hospital, where a diagnosis is made: an uncomplicated myocardial infarction (heart attack). He then spends the next 10 days recovering in the cardiac ward.

Until recently, this length of stay wasn't unusual in Canadian hospitals for an uncomplicated myocardial infarction. However, the clinically useful stay is estimated to be only five days. In other words, after the first 120 hours, the patient is no longer getting needed hospital care — he's essentially receiving hotel-like services.

Why isn't he discharged earlier to save money?

CASE STUDY 2

An older widow experiences recurring lower back problems. The pain is minor and manageable with aspirin, but the persistence is a source of annoyance. Her family physician orders an X-ray and, upon inspection, suggests that the pain is simply a result of "old age" and declares that nothing more can be done for it.

The woman isn't pleased and finds another doctor. She too suggests that not much can be done — the occasional painkiller is the best course of action. Still unconvinced, the woman finds a third doctor. This new physician runs various tests, prescribes a number of drugs, and schedules her for routine follow-ups. The pain doesn't subside under the new drug regimen, but the woman is delighted with the doctor's efforts. The attention is the highlight of the day. So she visits her new physician at least once a week.

Why is the physician acting as the widow's social companion?

CASE STUDY 3

A second-year university student aspires to get into the Faculty of Medicine. He hopes to follow in the footsteps of his father, an established surgeon.

In his first year of university, his grades were good but hardly top tier. As he enters the second year, he knows that his academic performance must improve despite the heavy course load.

In October, he begins to have powerful headaches. The family physician refers him to a neurologist, who works in the same hospital as the patient's father. After giving the student a quick examination, the neurologist suggests that the problem is little more than a tension headache, but to be safe he offers him an MRI scan. The student — aware that the best treatment might be dropping biochemistry and taking it over the summer — decides that it's better to be safe than sorry. He opts for the MRI scan, which reveals no problem.

Why does the student get the expensive and unnecessary test?

★   ★   ★

In each instance above, the medicare system has been misused. Why?

4.1 The Problem

"Then make the water flow uphill." So goes the punchline in a popular engineering joke. The joke isn't worth remembering, but perhaps the underlying point is: it may be possible to make water defy gravity, but doing so is hardly the basis of an efficient hydroelectric project — a common-sense rule that the failed engineers in the joke never do appreciate. Amazingly, it's this sort of common sense that our politicians seem unable to apply to the medicare system.

How do we make medicare more efficient? Governments have pondered the question for three decades now. The exercise is more than just intellectually interesting — as Canada's population grows older, the medicare system will need to become more cost effective or it will collapse. No wonder, then, that governments have appointed task forces, commissions, and panels to review the state of the system and recommend changes. Government reports on health care have become a cottage industry in Canada; between 1986 and 1993, for example, 13 major reports were issued.[1]

There have been so many reports that in 1991 the Canadian Medical Association, the Canadian Hospital Association, and the Canadian Nurses Association jointly published a book summarizing the various government reports. The book is now hopelessly outdated, and many newer reports have been produced.

A simple list of reports does little to reflect the incredible amount of time and energy required in drafting such a report. The National Forum on Health, for example, spent two and a half years reviewing Canada's health care system, at a cost of over $10 million. The price tag isn't surprising — the forum had a support staff of 31. They produced dozens of short reports, questionnaires, surveys, and even a video.

These major reports reflect only the tip of the iceberg; beneath the surface, there are tens of thousands of additional pages dedicated to the subject in the form of internal reports, studies, and position papers. And governments don't have a monopoly on health care analysis. Unions, professional associations, and consumer groups have all turned out their share of reports. Hundreds of conferences of doctors, nurses, deputy ministers, health economists, and policy analysts have discussed the issue at length. Even the Canadiana section at the local bookstore is littered with books on the topic.

There is, then, no shortage of work done on the medicare system. And, in all fairness, some practical ideas have arisen from all the analysis. Recommendations calling for greater hospital cooperation, stronger utilization of long-term-care facilities, cost-effective preventive medicine, better financial tracking systems, and other such initiatives are — in principle, anyway — worth considering.

A western libertarian once commented that the more paper bureaucrats turn out on an issue, the worse the situation becomes. The view is cynical but perhaps not completely unfair. As the years have passed, the volume of material on medicare has grown steadily, but medicare has noticeably worsened.

Ministers of health rarely last long in the portfolio. Consider Ontario. Over a 17-year period, 11 politicians have held the health portfolio in that province. And there have been seven deputy ministers. This turnover is all the more remarkable given that Ontario has had relative political stability during that period, with three majority governments.

Granted, not all provincial governments are created equal. Some have done better with the resources available, others worse. Still, health care is a hot issue in provincial politics from coast to coast, without regard for the political stripe of a particular government. Roy Romanow, the NDP premier of Saskatchewan, faces just as many harsh criticisms during Question Period over the closure of Regina's Plains Health Centre as his more conservative counterpart Mike Harris does in Ontario over the closure of Hamilton's Hotel Dieu.

It just doesn't seem to add up. On one side of the equation, governments have tremendous incentives to deal effectively with the health care issue. Add to those incentives the countless analyses of the system and the hundreds of recommendations made in various reports. Yet the result is completely off-track. Governments are trying increasingly aggressive regimens of treatment only to find that the patient still fades.

The problem is that the patient has been misdiagnosed. Governments are treating the symptoms of the disease, not the ailment itself. As a result a particular government initiative will sometimes produce the intended result (cost savings, greater efficiency, etc.) and sometimes not. Even the best treatments can only produce minor benefits. And, because of the incredible complexity of the system, all these experiments produce unintended side effects.

What, then, is the real diagnosis? Why is medicare failing?

The trouble with medicare is medicare itself. That is, the principles upon which the system rests doom it to failure. Today's reforms attempt to preserve the framework of the system and, by doing so, ensure that success will never be achieved. The efforts may be well intentioned — but so are the engineers in the joke who attempt to force water to flow uphill.

Here is what the Canadian experts miss: *the fundamental flaw of the medicare system is that patients bear no direct costs for the medical services they receive.*

4.2 The Patient as Consumer?

Are patients the problem with the health care system?

This question is based on the economic premise that a health care system balances supply (production) and demand (consumption): that is, there's a natural equilibrium between the services produced by physicians and other health care providers and the desire of patients to receive these services. With medicare — a publicly funded system in which there's no direct cost to the patient-consumer — demand naturally rises. Because patients needn't worry about cost, they can demand more medical services.

Canadians don't usually think about health care in this way. Perhaps on an intellectual level the argument is somewhat acceptable. It is well known that cost influences the balance between supply and demand. If the local grocery store puts apples on sale, shoppers will buy more apples — the lower the price, the higher the demand. Canadians know this from everyday experience. No one would suggest that a grocer wishing to sell more apples should double the price.

Economists describe this phenomenon as the law of demand. According to David Henderson, the law states that, "when the price of a good rises, the amount demanded falls, and when the price falls, the amount demanded rises." Indeed, "on this law is built almost the whole edifice of economics" (7). The law is so well accepted, notes Henderson, that "Nobel Laureate George Stigler responded years ago that if any economist found a true counterexample, he would be 'assured of immortality, professionally speaking, and rapid promotion.'" To date, there have been no counterexamples.

The Economics 101-style argument against medicare is frequently found in articles and essays. Opinion pieces in the *Financial Post*, whose authors can hardly be termed medicare supporters, use food as an analogy. The strategy is simple: Canadians understand from experience that the law of demand applies to the production and consumption of food, so such an analogy enables them to see that health care is the same. "Medicare is run . . . like a soup kitchen," explains one columnist about the woes of the health care system (Frum, "Reform"). Another writes that "health care has evolved into a Sunday brunch where consumers can feast on expensive items without concern for cost" (Gratzer, "Canadian"). In *Youthquake*, Ezra Levant forwards the most complete food-based argument:

> Now imagine that we all had to pay a Foodcare tax to the government every month and that, in return, each citizen gained unfettered access to restaurant service. Foodcare would be free and available equally to everyone in the country, regardless of ability to pay or need for nourishment, and run by selfless bureaucrats. . . . (88)

In other words, imagine if the government treated food as it does health care. Both are basic needs. Both are frequently consumed. What if the state financed both? Levant fills in the details:

The rest of the crazy story would be pretty easy to predict. With price no longer an object, Canadians wouldn't shop around for the best deals. Instead they would try for the biggest possible share of the restaurant pie. They'd eat out as much as they could stand.

Restaurants too would change. They wouldn't have to control costs or compete based on value for the dollar. After all, the government would pay for anything a customer wanted. The country would be swamped with T-bone steak buffets and caviar drive-throughs. (88)

Strong stuff. But is this analogy realistic? Can health care be overconsumed like free T-bone steaks and caviar? Levant's argument is eloquent. The problem is that Canadians don't see the provision of health care in terms of production and consumption.

Medical care has a mythical element to it. Part of this perception is rooted in societal values instilled in us as children. Mother — the centre of the universe for any youngster — looks to the physician for help. "Do what the doctor says" and "Don't worry, the doctor will make you feel better" every child is told. The mother's respect for the physician and, by extension, the health care profession, is passed on to the child as generational wisdom.

And the awe with which we view health care doesn't diminish as we grow up. We become increasingly aware of the fragility, wonder, and complexity of life. For this reason, doctors are greatly respected, and medicine is called "the noblest profession." Parents may dread the prospects of their children becoming rock musicians, but a physician in the family is always welcomed. Doctors, after all, save lives.

This description is slightly simplistic. Over the years, malpractice cases and instances of sexual misconduct have tarnished the overall reputation of the medical profession. Today patients respect the analyses of their physicians, but they don't accept them without critical thought — a strong contrast from the turn of the century. Nevertheless, the medical profession is held in high regard. If a man collapses in a crowded theatre, people instinctively react by calling out, "Is there a doctor in the house?" No one responds by saying, "That's all he needs: a heart attack and now a doctor." Doctors may no longer be beyond criticism, but as a group they are still respected.

All this fuels a rather misleading view of medicine and, as a result, health care. To Canadians, the term "health care" is equated with life-saving measures. "When Canadians think about health care," notes Bill

Robson of the C.D. Howe Institute, "they think about emergency rooms and emergency care." This image is reflected in our culture. Movies, television shows, and novels portray neurosurgeons performing groundbreaking surgeries or the busy work of emergency room physicians saving victims of car accidents. These extreme images are very different from personal experience. How many Canadians have ever been in a serious accident or have become candidates for complex brain surgery? Few. Instead, most Canadians have experienced the lazy pace of a dull walk-in clinic. Yet the extreme image holds.

Hence, Canadians don't think about supply and demand when they think about health care. Rather, they associate the term with life and death; it is deemed exceptional and unique.

Returning to the law of demand, we can easily see why the analogy just doesn't work. Widow Jones is a frugal shopper and would certainly buy more apples (or, as Levant suggests, T-bone steaks) when they go on sale, but does she really get more medical treatment because it's free? To carry the comparison to an extreme, does she endulge in MRI scans, blood tests, and barium enemas just because they're free? Each is hardly the sort of thing any rational person would do unless absolutely necessary. Just because Widow Jones has an unlimited health care budget doesn't mean she's a masochist. If free health care creates unnecessary demand, why don't we spend Saturday nights getting X-rays?

Health economist Robert Evans underscores this point when he writes that "the common description of health care [is] as a need. . . . [This is] different from ordinary commodities for which . . . wants, when backed by willingness to pay, become demands" (53). The key word is "need." Evans illustrates the point: "The statement 'Oh Lord, I need a Mercedes-Benz' is a joke. 'Oh Lord, I need a coronary artery bypass graft!' isn't" (53).

Economics professor Ake Blomqvist summarizes this view nicely (though he doesn't agree with it):

> Whether or not economic analysis can make a significant contribution to explaining the rise in health expenditure depends a great deal on the degree of choice that society has in providing health services. Those who don't think there is much, argue somewhat as follows: "At a given time, with given medical technology, . . . there is a 'best' treatment to which a person with a particular health problem is entitled. Given technology, the doctor has little choice with respect to recommending or not recommending

hospitalization for whatever length of time, performing or not performing surgery, and with respect to type of medication he prescribes. Similarly, he has little or no choice with respect to performing or ordering diagnostic tests of different kinds for a given patient, and so on." (2–3)

By this line of reasoning, health care is understood to be a need. Widow Jones may *want* a T-bone steak, but she doesn't need it. However, she may well *need* a coronary artery bypass graft — without the surgery, she will die. The matter appears to be settled. A very complicated issue has clarified itself. Common sense dictates that health care can't be overconsumed. There's little left to be done besides some cleaning up — cancelling the *Financial Post* subscription and returning *Youthquake* to the bookstore for a refund.

So the concept of overconsumption seems implausible — people don't choose to get sick, and treatments are rarely pleasant. Need (rather than demand) in health care doesn't seem to rise just because there's no cost. A patient suffering from a disease must be treated regardless of whether the medical services are paid out of pocket or by the state. Following this argument, it makes sense to keep health care free, because people will consume only as much of it as they need. Such thinking is certainly not confined to noneconomists or even to Canadians. In 1971, for example, a scholar testified before a U.S. Senate committee that demand in health care wouldn't rise if costs were eliminated (Newhouse and the Insurance Experiment Group 3).

Some supporters of medicare make a further point: maybe it's possible for price to influence demand in health care, but such a situation isn't beneficial. Take the overzealous father whose daughter develops a high fever. In a free system, he won't hesitate to rush his child to the emergency room at 3 a.m. If his daughter only has a flu, the trip has been wasteful. The father probably should have just called the pediatrician in the morning. But what if his daughter has meningitis? Then the trip has been well justified — a few hours can make the difference between life and death. From society's point of view, it's better to have 10 overzealous fathers rushing their mildly sick daughters into emergency rooms rather than one father who is deterred by price. In the latter scenario, the father will deprive his daughter of needed care. Society plays it safe with a free health care system — people may overuse some basic services, but major illnesses (and major expenses) can be reduced.

In *Universal Health Care*, the Armstrongs draw on the work of several Canadian experts to argue both points.[2] They conclude that

Fees do not work to appropriately allocate care primarily because the "laws" of supply and demand do not work here. The theory of supply and demand rests on the assumption of readily available choices, alternatives, and information. For the most part, people don't have a choice about when, if, where, [or] how to get sick or become disabled. . . . (45)

There are, then, two separate and powerful arguments against the supply-demand model of health care.

1. Patients don't demand health care; they need it. Price is thus irrelevant.
2. Although use may be greater in a free system, the preventive aspects of the increased use result in lower overall expenditures.

Does supply and demand work with health care? Many disputes — particularly hotly debated moral issues — stem from differences in belief. No amount of argument will resolve these disputes. Neither side in the abortion debate is able to prove that its beliefs are right. Fortunately, the health care issue is possible to resolve — consumption is a question of applied economics, not morality. Either price influences the consumption of health care services or it doesn't.

In the 1960s and 1970s, several economists attempted to determine whether user fees really affect consumption. These studies focused on hospital stays (Feldstein), physician and hospital expenses (Rosett-Huang), and other aspects of health care, such as office visits and hospital admissions (Phelps-Newhouse).[3] Unfortunately, they used nonexperimental data — the economists drew their data from historical sources, thereby affecting the validity of the experiments. Not surprisingly, the results of the studies differed. "Perhaps the only agreement in the literature by the mid-1970s," notes Phelps, "was that 'price mattered'" (qtd. in Ramsay, "Medical" 22). And there was a larger problem with these studies. The attempt to look at user fees on consumption — price elasticity of demand, as the economists called it — in no way determined the wellness of those involved.

The California-based RAND think tank set out to resolve these issues. It tapped the expertise of some of the top scholars in the world to design an experiment that would measure (1) the effects of price on consumption, and (2) the health of those involved (health outcome). The RAND Health Insurance Experiment proved to be one of the largest and longest running social science research projects ever completed. Headed by Harvard professor Joseph P. Newhouse, it involved approximately 2,000 nonelderly families and ran from 1974 to 1982. The cost was a staggering $136 million (1984 US dollars).

The most interesting aspect of the experiment involved the use of medical services (additional work was done on dental and mental health services). Families were assigned two fundamentally different types of health insurance: a *free-care plan* and a *user-fee plan*. Those with the free-care plan paid no out-of-pocket expenses; visits to the family physician were as free as a visit to the emergency room. Those with the user-fee plan paid a certain percentage of cost up to a maximum of $1,000, depending on family income.

The experiment serves as an excellent test of the influence of price on health care demand. If health care isn't influenced by price, there should be no difference in expenditures between the free-care group and the user-fee group. But if price does influence demand, expenditures should be lower for the user-fee group, because they face a cost every time they use a service — if they want to save money, they must forgo some health care services, such as a visit to the doctor.

What did RAND find? "Use of medical services responds unequivocally to changes in the amount paid out of pocket" (Newhouse and the Insurance Experiment Group 40). It turns out that individual expenses in the free-care plan were significantly higher than those in the user-fee plan. Expenses were 45% higher for the free-care individuals over those who had high user fees up to $1,000.[4]

Comparing the free-care group with the user-fee group, RAND found that in any given year the free-care people were more likely

- to use medical services (28% more often),
- to see a physician more regularly (67% more visits), and
- to get admitted to a hospital (30% more often).

The RAND Health Insurance Experiment had several groups with differing user fees. Even when people paid a rather small user fee (25% of total costs), there was a noticeable drop in health expenditures: 10% less than the free plan. *Price influences demand.*

There's still one unresolved issue: what effect did user fees have on the health of these individuals? They used fewer medical services, but were they sicker as a result? Again the conclusion was unequivocal: "Our results show that the . . . increase in services had little or no measurable effect on health status for the average adult" (243). Those with the free-care plan used far more services, at far greater expense, without improving their overall health. In addition, there was no significant difference between the two groups in the risk of dying or measures of pain and worry. The RAND researchers noted that in only one instance did the free-care plan have benefits over the user-fee plans: for the poor with high blood pressure. The authors conclude, however, that "a one-time screening examination achieved most of the gain in blood pressure that free care achieved" (243).

Curiously, individuals on the free-care plan seemed to be less productive members of society. They experienced 20% more days per year of restricted activity and 13% more days per year of work loss than the individuals with high user fees (see chapter 6 of *Free for All?*). Both groups, however, reported the same overall satisfaction with their health care.

We can draw a few conclusions from these results.

- Health care consumption is influenced by price.
- Health outcome isn't (within reason). In other words, when people are put on a free-care plan, they overconsume health care. And the resulting difference in expenditures is large.
- People are able to accurately judge their own health needs. If provided with an incentive to economize, they can correctly determine when visiting a doctor is appropriate and when it is unnecessary.

The first two points settle the lingering dispute — it turns out that a supply-demand model does apply to health care. Thus, in a free system, overconsumption is possible with health care, as it is with food. Ezra Levant was right after all.

The third point has profound implications. It turns out that people do understand their own health needs. This realization is counter-intuitive. After all, people perceive medical care in a mythical light. How can an individual with no medical training understand his or her own needs? Very well, in fact. The much-touted preventive qualities of free health care prove to be imagined.

Given the RAND results, it's clear that the commonly held perceptions of health care are inaccurate. Associating health care with life-saving measures is hopelessly misleading. This is where the critics of supply-demand run aground — health care is vastly more than a team of ER doctors madly piecing together a car accident victim.

The use of economic terms may serve as a distraction. Let's attempt, then, to put the observations into a model. People generally think of health care in terms of life-saving measures. Were this model accurate, making health care "free" would have no effect on total cost. But, alas, the RAND experiment shows that it does. Despite your preconceived ideas about health care, your experiences with medicare probably support this claim. The odds are overwhelming that in the last five years, say, you didn't have delicate neurosurgery or a groundbreaking heart transplant. It's more likely that you saw a family physician on numerous occasions for minor complaints such as a bad flu.

A new model is in order: health care can be divided into life-saving services and non-life-saving services. Different experts have different phrases and terms to describe these categories. In *Who Shall Die?*, Victor Fuchs divides modern medicine according to the intended results: "curing" and "caring" (see 64–67). Economist Ake Blomqvist divides health care based on price:

> Even though most families have some medical expenses in a given year, the vast majority will spend less than five hundred dollars. . . . Furthermore, much of this expenditure will be incurred to deal with relatively minor and, in some cases, "discretionary" health problems: cuts and bruises, twisted ankles, bad colds or headaches, minor elective surgery, etc. . . . For the few individuals who have a major "serious" health problem, however, the cost may greatly exceed what they would be able to pay. . . . (16)

How Blomqvist and Fuchs distinguish types of health care — by price or by intended result — isn't nearly as important as the recognition that health care *can be* divided into two categories.

As a practical matter, the classifications used by Blomqvist and Fuchs aren't that different. An expensive service — a catastrophic expenditure, as Blomqvist would term it — is likely to be curative, whereas a service meant to deal with a discretionary problem is largely "caring," by Fuchs's definition. Using such a model, it's possible to see that medicine is more than a basic need.

Consider a seven-year-old girl with a throat infection. The doctor examines her throat and notes the bacterial infection. There are three options.

1. Do nothing. The girl's natural defences will probably clear up the infection in a week.
2. Prescribe general antibiotics. The infection will subside in four days.
3. Prescribe powerful, specific antibiotics. The infection will end in three days.

There's no difference between the three options. In each case, the bacteria is defeated. However, from the girl's point of view, the third option is greatly preferable, for suffering will be minimized. Of course, this option comes at a price. Drugs aren't free. The cost of the antibiotics is modest, and the convenience is great. And convenience, not life itself, is the goal of the treatment. Childhood is filled with many similar examples — penicillin to treat a sore throat, amoxicillin to clear an ear infection. We forget how little these treatments have to do with curing and how much they have to do with caring.

But it's easy to draw another common scenario in which the convenience isn't so great and the cost is much higher. Consider another seven-year-old girl with a throat infection. This time, the father is less worried about his daughter's throat and more annoyed by the string of infections, visits to the doctor, and antibiotics. He asks the physician if something can be done. The doctor responds by proposing a tonsillectomy (removal of the tonsils). The father agrees, and the surgery is scheduled. The measure isn't necessary for the girl's well-being. Calculating the one-night stay in the hospital, the cost of the operating room, and other expenses, the convenience — more for the father than his daughter — becomes an expensive proposition.

Pediatric tonsillectomy for convenience can be added to a long list of such services. In a free system, there is no incentive to think twice about consulting a doctor over minor ailments or staying longer in a hospital after surgery.

The argument about convenience can be expanded. It's more convenient, for example, to see a doctor in the middle of the night with a sore wrist than to wait until morning. As a result, some people go to the emergency room at 3 a.m. with such minor ailments — hardly life-and-death situations. A sore wrist isn't even an emergency per se. For the patient, there is convenience; for the system, there is cost. A consultation in the emergency room can run over $100. A visit to the family physician is under $20. In a free system — one in which patients see no connection between the costs of the services they receive and the amounts they pay in taxes — the only apparent difference between these visits is convenience.

Convenience, of course, can take another form: providing the patient with peace of mind. A diagnostic test may be run simply to allay a patient's irrational fears. Until restrictions were imposed, many patients would request a yearly cholesterol blood test even though they had no history of problems and no risk factors. Why, then, did they want the test? When the effects of high cholesterol on health were prominently featured in the media, people worried about their cholesterol levels. Faced with a choice between a free test and the ongoing worry, they decided on the test — and thus on peace of mind.

Patients, then, have an incentive to overconsume in a "free" system. In terms of the model of health care outlined above, the non–life-saving aspects of health care present opportunities for excessive utilization by consumers. Put another way, such health care acts like a commodity. The potential to overconsume for the sake of convenience is consistent with this statement. The results of the RAND Health Insurance Experiment illustrate the point. But logical clarity is one thing; convincing evidence is quite another. Is there strong evidence of overconsumption in the Canadian health care system?

There is a simple — and perhaps simplistic — argument to this effect. If, in a free system, demand increases and people overconsume, then expenditures should rise, with a modest change in overall results. Applying this argument to medicare, health expenditures should rise, but the overall health of the population should stay the same. In fact, Canada's health spending nearly doubled between the mid-1980s and the mid-1990s, but there was no evidence that people were healthier as a result (Foot and Stoffman 172).

The argument has its problems. In addition to an increase in demand, various factors can contribute to the rise in expenditures: an aging population, widespread staff unionization, and advances in medical technology, for example. Likely all four factors are responsible for higher expenditures. (The factors might be interrelated. For example, aging citizens are expensive in a free system because they demand more services.)

Rather than rely on crude indicators such as life expectancy, we should focus on patterns of usage. If, indeed, "free" health care translates into overconsumption, then we would expect that after the introduction of medicare

- the demand for medical services increased dramatically,
- the demand changed in nature, and
- the demand for services to address insignificant complaints developed.

This is, in fact, what happened.

*   *   *

Increased Demand

- In 1977, the Joint Advisory Committee of the Government of Ontario and the Ontario Medical Association reviewed usage within the medicare system and concluded with worry that "demand for medical care appears infinite" (32).
- In the five years before the introduction of medicare, physicians' incomes were 34% above the average for other professionals. In the five years after the introduction of medicare, physicians' incomes rose dramatically — to a full 47% above that of other professionals (Michael Walker, "Why" 4). The income increased even though the average work day shortened and the number of physicians per capita rose.

Altered Demand

- In 1973, the *New England Journal of Medicine* published an article on medical care in Quebec before and after the introduction of medicare (Enterline et al., "Distribution"). The article described a brief study of patients' behaviour. Medicare was new at the time, but the authors noted that, although physicians were contacted by patients with a similar frequency, the nature of the contacts had changed. Before medicare, patients often phoned physicians with minor problems (such calls weren't billed). But after the introduction of medicare, phone calls dropped, and face-to-face contacts increased by the same percentage. In other words, patients realized that the free phone call wasn't as satisfying as the (now) free personal contact.

Petty Demand

- Another article in the *New England Journal of Medicine* (Enterline et al., "Effects") reported the results of a survey of physicians in Quebec about the usage of the health care system before and after the introduction of medicare. Physicians believed that the number of frivolous patient complaints had increased by nearly 75%.
- According to the Ontario Task Force on the Use and Provision of Medical Services, Ontario physicians billed $200 million in 1990 for "treating" the common cold.

*   *   *

Medicare did increase the demand for health care. With free services, a scratchy throat is suddenly cause to see an ear-nose-throat specialist; a common cold is reason enough to visit the local walk-in clinic; a stress headache warrants a battery of tests; the aches and pains of old age need to be checked out by the geriatrician; and a sprained ankle is an "urgent" medical problem treated in an emergency room.[5]

But how often are emergency rooms, for instance, misused? The Saskatchewan Health Services Utilization and Research Commission concluded that nonurgent use is "a universal phenomenon" (1). In 1997, the Regina Health District found that from 43% to 49% of the ER patients at its three hospitals were nonurgent cases.

In *Patient Power! The Smart Patient's Guide to Health Care*, a family physician (with 25 years of experience) and a nurse write about the overconsumption of health care in a fictionalized — though realistic — conversation between two frustrated medical students:

> "I'm so sick of patients demanding a CT scan or an MRI for a tension headache. Most of the time they don't even know what they're asking for. All they know is that they read about it in a magazine and that we have the equipment here. If people only knew how many of these patients are getting those unnecessary tests because they're demanding them themselves." . . .
>
> "Yeah, I remember when I was doing my Family Medicine rotation, I thought I'd scream if one more person came into the office with a head cold. No matter how many times I said that there really wasn't anything I could do for them except tell them to go home and drink lots of fluids, they still demanded to be treated." (Parsons and Parsons 153)

The authors go on to describe a familiar situation in which a patient demands an unnecessary service:

> A young, pregnant woman walks into her doctor's office demanding a repeat ultrasound. The doctor looks at her chart and sees that the ultrasound the patient has already had was unequivocally normal and that the fetal growth was progressing as expected. Questioning reveals that the woman's husband had not been able to attend the first ultrasound and that the hospital [had] failed to provide her with a picture — and she wants one for her husband. (153–54)

The authors note the waste to the system. The test is medically unnecessary, and the demand is wasteful. They unhappily report that "this does, however, happen" (154).

And it does. In a system with no connection between usage and cost, convenience and peace of mind will inevitably become higher priorities. And they tie in to the present woes of the medicare system. After all, if patients in a free system tend to overconsume, then it's no surprise that medicare is so expensive and inefficient.

There are two ways in which a free system distorts consumption: the extent to which patients demand health care, and the type of care they demand.

The examples cited above largely focus on the additional usage of health care. Patients in a free system see physicians more frequently, they elect to get more tests, and they demand more treatments. A point only briefly touched on above — one worthy of greater exploration — is the *type* of service utilization in a free system. When cost isn't a consideration, patients utilize health services differently.

The proliferation of walk-in clinics and the abuse of emergency rooms fit the general pattern. A visit to a walk-in clinic or an emergency room for a minor complaint may be very expensive to the system as opposed to seeing a family physician, but the patient has all the gain without the cost.

In a free system, people will tend to demand the most expensive services — they will look for the best-trained providers and the most impressive and convenient facilities — whether or not their condition warrants them. The resulting trend away from cost effectiveness has hopelessly influenced the development of medicare over the years.

4.3 Providing the Care: Doctors in Medicare

In a free health care system, demand increases significantly — enough that experts have even suggested that demand becomes "infinite" (Joint Advisory Committee 32). The implications of this observation on usage are profound. Equally profound are the effects on supply. Doctors, it follows logically, will do well under such a system (at least until billings are restricted).

Consider a family physician with a suburban office. Under a "free" system, many patients are likely to see her with minor — even frivolous — problems. If a patient comes in with the common cold, the doctor is quickly able to conclude that nothing can be done. An experienced physician would probably be able to examine the patient and make the diagnosis in under five minutes. The visit is short, uncomplicated, and financially rewarding. Such a visit will earn the physician about $15. Now imagine if the physician sees just four such patients a day. The annual compensation would be around $15,000. The excess demand in the system created by the lack of direct cost is very beneficial to the providers. It's not surprising, then, that a Saskatchewan study found that family physicians spend 10% of their time dealing with patients complaining of cold and flu symptoms.

In fact, if demand is "infinite," doctors have less need to worry about satisfying patients' whims — there will always be more patients. It's not coincidental that after the introduction of medicare physicians basically stopped doing house calls. Similarly, physicians soon stopped listing their home phone numbers in telephone directories.

And if demand is "infinite," physicians have little difficulty making a decent living — even in areas where there are many doctors. In 1979, Ake Blomqvist used statistics provided by the Canadian Medical Association to show that no relationship existed between the number of physicians per capita in a province and a physician's income. In fact, Blomqvist noted, if any conclusion can be drawn from the analysis, it is that the fewer patients a physician has, the higher his or her income (101).

There are two points we can draw from Blomqvist's work. (1) *Patient demand is so high that physicians aren't in competition with one another.* Generally, an increase in the number of providers results in greater competition and, as a result, a drop in average income. So, for example, the more restaurants there are in downtown Toronto, the harder it will be to turn a profit. Blomqvist's analysis indicates that competition between physicians doesn't occur. A look at physicians in urban centres provides additional evidence. Consider that between 1971 and 1981 the number of general practitioners rose by 67% in Winnipeg, whereas the population grew by only 10% (Roch, Evans, and Pascoe 21). There was, then, a surge in supply, but the average physician's income didn't drop. This supports the assertion that the demand for health care is insatiable when patients don't face direct costs.

(2) *Physicians are often able to make as much money or even more money treating fewer patients (within limits).* This possibility suggests that patients' overconsumption of health care is profitable to physicians. But it also suggests that by looking only at the demand side of the equation, we misrepresent the situation somewhat. The supply side — that is, the physicians — may also influence utilization.

In a healthy doctor-patient relationship, the doctor offers medical advice and the patient decides what to accept based on health care needs and financial situation. Fees temper demand. As a result, patients ask themselves questions such as "Is this test really worth the expense?" or "Do I really need the surgery, or will pain management do?" Without having to pay any cost, the patient is willing to accept far more services, thereby distorting the balance.

But doctors are active participants in the resulting overconsumption. After all, they have a financial incentive to overprovide services. The natural check on this incentive is the patient's desire not to spend too much money for care. In a "free" system, this check doesn't exist.

Because physicians are compensated on a fee-for-service basis, they have an incentive to provide many services. But does this incentive really affect overall health costs?

Again, we can turn to the results of the RAND Health Insurance Experiment to shed light on the issue. The RAND think tank compared the health expenditures and outcomes of two different types of insurance holders: those with a free-care plan, and those with Health Maintenance Organization (HMO) type of coverage. Under either plan, people saw no direct costs for health care services. However, under the HMO system, the doctor was paid a flat rate by the insurance company, and under the free-care plan the physician was paid on a fee-for-service basis by the insurance company.

Doctors under the fee-for-service system thus had a financial incentive to overprovide, whereas HMO physicians didn't. The result: the expenditures in the free-care plan were 28% higher. The health outcomes, however, were comparable. The biggest differences were admissions and total hospital days — under the HMO system, both were 40% fewer (Newhouse and the Insurance Experiment Group 280).

The results compare closely with those of other studies. Again, it's relatively easy to see how physicians can provide more services for minor problems. They can do more follow-ups, for instance. But where does the oversupply end? After all, patients will never agree to certain procedures unless they are absolutely necessary. Major surgery, such as a hysterectomy, comes to mind.

It seems, however, that even surgeries are influenced by the fee-for-service system. An audit of medical services in California, for instance, discovered that when the compensation of a group of physicians changed from salary to fee for service, the number of hysterectomies increased fivefold (see Blomqvist 65–148). Other surgeries follow a similar pattern. Some physicians, for example, suggest that 75% of all tonsil-lectomies are unnecessary (Blomqvist 87).

This pattern seems somewhat unbelievable at first. Tonsillectomies are one thing, but hysterectomies? After all, a hysterectomy is a major operation with a lengthy recovery period — surely no woman wants to undergo the surgery unless it's absolutely necessary. It seems logical to assume that the operation either is or is not necessary. But usually there are many options available for treatment. Consider a patient suf-fering from excessive menstruation as a result of noncancerous fibroid tumours.[6] She can choose no treatment, removal of the tumours, or removal of the entire uterus (a hysterectomy). However, if the doctor is paid by the service, he or she may well push the hysterectomy option harder. This is a physician-manufactured demand.

A Canadian study published in the *New England Journal of Medicine* supports this point (Dyck et al.). Between 1964 and 1971, the number of hysterectomies in Saskatchewan rose by 72.1%, whereas the number of women over the age of 15 increased by 7.2%. The Ministry of Health, alarmed by the trend, asked the College of Physicians and Surgeons to investigate. When this body began monitoring the situation for "unjus-tified" procedures, the number of surgeries dropped dramatically. Between 1970 and 1974, the number of hysterectomies in the province dropped by 32.8% (1326).

There's further evidence that the introduction of medicare allowed physicians to create greater demand for their services. In 1979, Blomqvist prepared an analysis of "elective" surgical procedures for each province over a two-year period (see 101–02). He analysed the number of proce-dures per capita against the number of physicians. The result: of the 28 procedures, 23 showed a statistically significant correlation between the number of physicians and the number of procedures. For example, for every 1% increase in surgeons per capita, the number of gall bladder surgeries rose by 1.06%. Elective surgeries to the middle ear, nose and sinuses, hernias, hemorrhoids, prostates, and joints all showed dramati-cally higher frequency when the number of surgeons rose in a particu-lar geographic area.

An article published in the *Canadian Journal of Economics* in 1973 found a similar result. The authors reasoned that, if demand genera-tion by physicians didn't exist, "a 1 percent increase in physician stock (per capita) should lead to a 1 percent decrease in workload and gross receipts per physician," with the total number of services per person remaining unchanged (Evans, Parish, and Scully 389). In fact, the number of physicians did have a substantial impact on the volume of health care services. The elasticity of total services provided in response to an increase in the number of physicians was 0.85, not zero (389).

It is difficult, of course, to simply look at elective surgical procedures and the number of surgeons and draw conclusions. Some would argue that in provinces with fewer surgeons (and thus fewer procedures), a large number of medical problems remain "untreated." The issue, then, is not overservicing but underservicing. But if the results are taken in the context of the RAND experiment, this doesn't seem to be the case. Rather, doctors have a financial incentive to provide many services and therefore do so.

There are, of course, many ways in which doctors can offer more services than required. In addition to excessive surgical treatments, they can order many follow-up visits for basic illnesses. Sandra, a university student from Hamilton, recently moved to Winnipeg. When her prescription for a basic drug ran out, she went to a young family physician not far from her apartment. The physician asked her a few questions and then represcribed the drug to last a month. She advised Sandra to return in a month for a follow-up. "We'll make sure the medication is working properly," the doctor suggested. A month later, Sandra returned and, after a few questions, was prescribed the same medication — again only enough to last her a month. Clearly, the doctor was profiting from this arrangement. Each time Sandra returned for a refill, the doctor could charge the medicare system.

Such examples aren't rare. Doctors, after all, have to find ways to make money. Not every doctor, of course, is only interested in the bottom line, but as Sue Blevins, a retired nurse who has practised in both Canada and the United States, observes, "in a fee-for-service system, you're always looking for ways to bill."

Hence, a healthy man in his twenties is given annual checkups; a patient suffering from high blood pressure sees his doctor once a week for a quick blood pressure check; an older man goes to a walk-in clinic to have his ears cleaned. In each example, a patient receives a service that is hardly required. Annual checkups for a young man are excessive, as are weekly blood pressure checks. And the older man can probably be taught to clean his own ears.

Under a "free" system, it's not just patients who act in a counterproductive manner. The piper, to use an old cliché, calls the tune — and with health care, the piper is the payer. Because patients don't pay for the health care they receive, doctors end up serving the payer (the provincial fee schedule). The doctor-patient relationship is replaced by a doctor-payer relationship.

Doctors, then, are financially rewarded for maximizing the number of patients they see (and, for that matter, the number of tests and treatments they perform), and they are financially penalized for taking time to explain to their patients treatment options and preventive measures. In Ontario, many were shocked when it was reported that over 200 family physicians had billed the government for more than $400,000 each in 1994–95 (Bohuslawsky, "Patient Overdose"). These high-billing doctors had pushed through an average of 67 patients a day, or one every eight minutes. Members of the doctors' communities may have been surprised by the story, but the doctors' bankers weren't.

4.4 Medicare's Bogeyman

It's remarkable how much time some people spend criticizing the group they believe is most responsible for medicare's problems. Some experts blame the physicians, while others blame the patients. Such conclusions are usually drawn along ideological lines.

Right-wing politicians and policy analysts tend to think that patients are the main culprit. Thus, a conservative writer (and former Conservative MP) such as Patrick Boyer or a fiscal conservative such as Ralph Klein are content to look at demand in the system.

Left-leaning experts are more concerned with the physicians. In *Second Opinion: What's Wrong with Canada's Health-Care System and How to Fix It*, Dr. Michael Rachlis and Carol Kushner (a former union consultant) spend an entire chapter pinning blame on physicians for the system's woes. As if out of guilt over their overwhelming criticism of doctors, they write in their introduction that "this isn't a doctor-bashing book; instead it might be described as a hard critical look at medicine and the health care system" (x).

The solutions that these analysts then recommend follow from their political perspectives. On the right, user fees are usually advocated; on the left, flat compensation for providers (i.e., salary rather than fee for service) is often recommended.

Yet finger pointing — at either physicians or patients — misses the point somewhat. There is no one medicare bogeyman, easily identifiable and notoriously evil. Rather, the problem lies in the fact that the doctor-patient relationship has been corrupted by the "free" nature of the system. As a result, both doctors and patients act in undesirable ways. Patients choose to overconsume, and doctors tend to overprovide.

To understand how to create a more efficient health care system, it's important for us to understand what's awry with the present arrangement. Meaningful solutions to the problems of the system will be discussed in chapters 6 and 7, but first we need to recognize the real roots of the problems; vilifying doctors or patients accomplishes little.

4.5 The Institutional Providers

"Appropriate, effective, and efficient." With these three words, the members of the Health Services Utilization Working Group summarized the way in which Canada's hospital sector ought to work (9). Yet the group of 11 prominent health care policy analysts concluded in their 1994 paper for the Conference of Federal/Provincial/Territorial Deputy Ministers of Health that, in fact, our hospital system falls desperately short of achieving these three basic criteria. No wonder, then, that their report concludes by calling for "significant changes" (38).

This conclusion of the committee — all members were supportive of the medicare system but collectively disappointed in the hospital sector — wasn't a surprise. Provincial governments had been disillusioned with their hospitals for years. The consensus was that the hospitals were inappropriately used, ineffective at care delivery, and inefficient in resource use. But careful consideration of the hospital sector was more than an academic exercise, for hospitals are the single largest expense of every provincial health budget. Typically, they consume 40¢ of every provincial health dollar spent.

Hence, hospital reform has been the preoccupation of provincial governments for close to a decade (see Deber, Mhatre, and Baker for a detailed description). In 1992, for example, the Manitoba government released its report on the future of health care (see Government of Manitoba). At the time, Manitoba was struggling to contain health care costs in an attempt to balance the budget. And what was the most radical and far-reaching recommendation? A strategic shift in patient care away from the big teaching hospitals, the Health Sciences Centre and the St. Boniface Hospital, and toward lower-cost facilities.

The study noted that patient care costs $775 per day at the teaching hospitals but only $410 per day at smaller community hospitals such as Concordia. Long-term-care facilities were even cheaper at $276 per day. The report went one step further and suggested that for some patients home care and community-based programs would be even more cost effective than institutional care.

The thrust of the recommendation — that patient care is overly reliant on expensive institutional care — was a relatively hot topic in the early 1990s. Home care, for example, was one of the major topics discussed at the Fourth Canadian Conference on Health Economics at the University of Toronto in August 1990.

But few people stopped to ask the relevant questions. Why had the system become so reliant on institutional care? What incentives within the system distorted usage to this extent? Why was an elderly woman occupying a bed in the surgery ward at $775 a day when a home-care program would probably have been just as effective at under $100 a day?

The last question is particularly troubling, and it raises yet another question: how frequently does this situation occur? The Health Services Utilization Working Group's report, "When Less Is Better: Using Canada's Hospitals Efficiently," cites several studies that estimate inappropriate use at between 19% and 60% of total patient days, depending on the type of hospital (12). In other words, on any given day, roughly half the beds in a hospital are taken up by patients who don't need to be there. A recent study by the Manitoba Centre for Health Policy and Evaluation suggests that about 51% of hospital admissions are for nonacute care. A chart review involving over 1,095 patient days at Montreal's Royal Victoria Hospital found that 33% of these days were "inappropriate" and "non-medical" (Gagnon).

Why have hospitals, meant to provide acute care, become centres for nonacute care? Part of the answer lies with people's demands. Freed from financial obligation, patients want the best care. Given the choice between in-hospital recovery and day surgeries, people prefer the convenience of the hospital stay. Given the choice between a newer, impressive teaching hospital and an older, unimpressive community hospital, people choose the big centre.

But this is only part of the explanation. Hospitals, like other sectors of the medicare system, have been hopelessly influenced by government involvement. The reliance on institutional care is the result of years of government meddling in hospital care.

Before exploring the government's role, we should consider the four failings of the hospital sector.

1. *Redundancy*. Many hospitals provide the same services to the same areas. Despite the clear overlap, there's practically no cooperation between the institutions. As a result, money is squandered on redundant administration, separate purchasing, and unneeded services.

2. *Overutilization*. Studies have consistently shown that most hospital beds — intended to be used for active medical treatment — are used for nonacute care. Lower-cost methods of care should thus be employed.

3. *Unaccountability*. Although hospitals undergo basic financial auditing, few attempts have been made to determine the performance of the different institutions. Crude comparisons,[7] for example, suggest that not all hospitals are created equal.

4. *Ineffectiveness*. Occasionally covered in the media are horror stories of gross hospital mismanagement, such as the poor state of affairs at St. Michael's in Toronto (before its overhaul). Although such examples are rare, many hospitals are run in an unimaginative fashion, resisting innovation. Critics have long claimed that big savings could be achieved by streamlining administrations, prioritizing resources, and ending wasteful bureaucratic procedures.

There has been little investigation of the last point. The Fraser Institute, however, did compare hospital wages with their equivalents in the private sector. The study's authors reason that "Many jobs in hospitals are similar to jobs performed in other sectors of the economy. The largest overlap of comparable workers is between the hospital and hotel sectors" (Ramsay et al. 153). Thus, the wage comparisons were made between the unionized workers at the Royal Columbian Hospital and the unionized workers of the Greater Vancouver Hotel Union. "Many jobs, of course, cannot be compared directly, such as those in the hospital sector that require specific medical knowledge: this group includes people such as nurses, technicians, and lab assistants" (154). The study, then, excluded these special workers and compared 18 comparable occupations.

The results are surprising. A hotel plumber, for example, earns on average $15.21 per hour. At a hospital, a plumber earns $23.88. Table 4.1 lists some of the other wage comparisons (155).

TABLE 4.1

Unionized Hospital and Hotel Wages

Worker Type	Hospital Hourly Wage ($)	Average Hotel Hourly Wage ($)
Cleaner	15.93	12.51
Laundry Aide	16.67	12.40
Storekeeper	17.46	12.83
Cook 1	16.88	13.10
Maintenance Worker	18.04	13.89
Electrician	24.58	15.08
Painter	21.83	13.37
Switchboard Clerk	16.31	12.85

The comparison includes only 372 of the 766 (medically) nontechnical workers at the Royal Columbian Hospital. Given that the wage difference was $3.94 an hour, health economist Cynthia Ramsay extrapolates that the potential savings if all workers were paid the private sector equivalent would be in the order of $5.4 million per year — or about four percent of the hospital's annual salary expenditure. Assuming that other hospitals could save four percent on their total annual spending, the province would have $115 million more each year (154).

Over the years, some hospitals have made (small) steps toward addressing these problems. Hospitals in Metro Toronto formed a joint purchasing committee to capitalize on bulk purchasing. The Victoria Hospital and University Hospital in London voluntarily agreed to merge into the London Health Sciences Centre, thereby reducing the administrative overlap. In Sault Ste. Marie, a consolidation reduced 14 vice-presidential positions to five. In Newfoundland, seven hospitals (known as the St. John's Health Care Corporation) joined forces with a private company to operate a new central kitchen.

The problems with the present hospital system have been caused by two separate government actions. *First, the construction boom* — there are simply too many hospitals offering too many similar services, dating back to 1948, when the federal government offered the provinces a generous cost-sharing arrangement for the construction of new hospitals, under the National Health Grant Program. Over the next 12 years, the number of hospital beds in Canada grew at a rate double that of the population expansion. The program had triggered a hospital construction boom — one that would last for nearly three decades.

Part of the motivation for the construction craze was benevolent. It was widely believed that Canada's population would continue to grow well past the end of the century. Politicians believed that a large health care infrastructure was needed for that growth.

But there was also a more self-interested motivation — politicians of the day discovered a very good deal. With the National Health Grant Program, provincial politicians were able to get all the political benefits of constructing a new hospital at a fraction of the full cost. As Anne Crichton et al. note in *Health Care: A Community Concern?*, "backbenchers lobbied for hospitals to be built in their own constituencies — for at that time hospitals were a major symbol of caring and they brought jobs to an area" (9). Hospital construction, then, was as much the result of perceived need as of political opportunism.

The construction boom dominated the 1950s. Hospitals began dotting the landscape. And while the provinces were eagerly engaged in building, relatively little attention was paid to practical considerations, resulting in an overbuilt and inefficient system. Duncan Gordon, former chair of Toronto's Hospital for Sick Children, summarized the situation well when he noted,

> Look at the number of communities we have in Canada that have a Catholic hospital on one block and a Protestant one on the next. Each trying to outdo the other, to keep its grip on the community. No one ever questioned whether a town of 50,000 really needed two hospitals. (qtd. in Rachlis and Kushner, *Second Opinion* 50)

Second, the global budget — under the medicare system, patients don't directly pay for the services they receive. As a result, the provincial governments fund hospitals. Most provinces fund their hospitals through direct grants that cover all operational expenses — so-called global budgets. Such funds aren't tied to patient load or service delivery or, in fact, any set of performance indicators; rather, they are awarded according to the perceived need of individual hospitals to service their respective communities.

Global budget grants create several problems. For one thing, the budgeting is based on a "spend it or lose it" methodology. If a hospital has money left over at the end of a fiscal year, the amount is taken off the following year's grant. In other words, hospitals are encouraged to be wasteful. They are often financially penalized for selling dated or redundant equipment by having the following year's grant docked by the amount earned.

The most significant problem with global budgets is that they create no financial incentive for hospitals to service patients efficiently. If anything, such budgets create a disincentive — a well-run hospital that serves patients in a timely and cost-effective manner will see more patients, not more money.

To make matters worse, hospitals are indirectly rewarded for treating low-needs patients. After all, a patient suffering from, say, a minor dermatological problem will require little more than basic "hotel" services — food and laundry. On the other hand, high-needs patients, such as a patient recovering from a major heart attack, will require constant supervision, expensive drugs, and diagnostic tests. Because the administrator is given a fixed global budget, the clear preference is to "bed block" — that is, to fill beds with low-needs patients so that the expensive patients will have to be treated at another institution.

4.6 The City of Angels

Much of this chapter has focused on the incentives within the medicare system for those involved to make the wrong choices. Where these incentives exist, deviant results will be produced. This is a complicated way of phrasing a simple concept: if there are advantages in abusing a system, some people will.

Yet there are many patients who don't misuse the system. They go to a doctor only when they think it's necessary. Likewise, many physicians realize that the resources of the system are limited. They do everything they can to ensure that money isn't wasted, even if it means that they bill less. One particularly conscientious family physician explained to a group of first-year medical students that "there is only so much money in the system. The more unnecessary tests you order, the more nurses lose their jobs." But many people do abuse the system. No wonder — they have incentives to do so.

In the City of Angels, free health care isn't misused. Angels, after all, are a decent lot. An angel will only go to the doctor if absolutely necessary — no angel would dream of going to a physician with a cold. And angels don't get unnecessary tests or treatments. Similarly, no angel-doctor would ever think about providing unneeded services. Angels are good that way.

But what works in the City of Angels won't necessarily work for us. *And here's the real problem with medicare — it expects that people will act like angels.* We're no angels.

It's poor planning to design a system in which people have incentives to misuse it yet expect that they won't.

A good system — whether for a sector of the economy, such as health care, or for the entire economy itself — should be based on human nature. Such a system provides productive incentives so that individuals' actions benefit not only themselves but also the system as a whole. These systems aren't built for angels. Their aims may not be as noble, but these systems do work.

4.7 The Cynic's List of Perverse Incentives

At this point, we can put together a list of all the incentives within the medicare system for the various players: patients, doctors, hospital administrators, and politicians.

For the Patient

- Patients have an incentive to use the emergency room as the 24-hour office of a family physician. *Emergency rooms are convenient.*
- Patients have an incentive to run to the walk-in clinic for every minor ailment, including the common cold. *Walk-in clinics are easily accessible, and the consultation is fast.*
- Patients have an incentive to recover from surgeries in hospitals as opposed to undergoing day surgeries. *Recovery is more convenient in a hospital setting.*
- Patients have an incentive to get every diagnostic test for even the most minor complaints. *Tests provide peace of mind.*
- Patients have an incentive to stay in the hospital for lengthy periods of time. *Hospital care is easier than self-care.*
- Patients have an incentive to see many doctors about the same problem. *Many opinions are better than just one.*
- Patients have an incentive to have every ache and pain of old age checked out. *Aches and pains of old age require no treatment, but attention is nice.*
- Patients, even though young and healthy, have an incentive to see their doctors for annual checkups. *Frivolous checkups ease a hypochondriac's concerns.*

For the Doctor

- Doctors have an incentive to see as many patients as possible. *In a fee-for-service system, more services mean more fees.*
- Doctors have an incentive to order many tests. *Tests make diagnoses easier and keep patients happy.*
- Doctors have an incentive to see healthy patients frequently. *Visits from healthy patients make for healthy incomes.*
- Doctors have an incentive not to treat complicated cases. *Complicated cases are rarely compensated in an adequate manner.*
- Doctors have an incentive to treat minor illnesses. *Minor illnesses are easy to treat, and they pay well.*
- Doctors have an incentive to leave the country for greener pastures. *High incomes are highly tempting.*
- Doctors have an incentive to overservice patients with surgical procedures. *Surgery pays well.*
- Doctors have an incentive not to discuss treatment options and promote healthy living. *Billing schedules don't compensate for conversation.*

For the Health Care Administrator

- Health care administrators have an incentive not to cooperate with those of other hospitals. *Cooperation reduces global budgets and infringes on managers' autonomy.*
- Health care administrators have an incentive to introduce new, redundant services. *Expansion increases global budgets.*
- Health care administrators have an incentive to fill beds with low-needs patients. *Bed blocking reduces demand on global budgets.*
- Health care administrators have an incentive to negotiate rigid contracts with unions representing orderlies, food workers, and other support staff. *Contractual limitations help to enlarge global budgets.*
- Health care administrators have an incentive to produce excessive rules that slow down decision making. *Bureaucracies need administrators.*
- Health care administrators have an incentive not to contract services out. *Fewer services require fewer administrators.*
- Health care administrators have an incentive to limit government restructuring efforts. *Restructuring kills administrative jobs.*

For the Politicians

- Politicians have an incentive not to close redundant hospitals. *Closures are politically unpopular.*
- Politicians have an incentive not to clash with health care administrators, unions, and doctors. *Disagreements make poor public spectacles.*
- Politicians have an incentive not to change the system. *Medicare is popular.*
- Politicians have an incentive to make cost-cutting decisions for short-term budgetary gain that result in higher costs in the long term. *Short-term gains reflect short-term reality: the next election is always just around the corner.*
- Politicians have an incentive to allow waiting lists to develop. *Some type of cost control must occur.*
- Politicians have an incentive not to invest in high-tech diagnostic equipment. *MRI and CT scanners are expensive to buy and run.*
- Politicians have an incentive to limit a patient's ability to seek services. *The availability of health services must be limited in the name of cost control.*
- Politicians have an incentive to limit a doctor's ability to practise medicine. *The doctor-patient relationship is important, but saving money is more important.*
- Politicians have an incentive not to collect systemic information. *Information on waiting lists and mortality rates is damning.*
- Politicians have an incentive to allocate resources to better service the government's voter base. *Politicized medicine has political results.*

★ ★ ★

Returning to the three case studies described at the beginning of the chapter, we can consider each misuse of the medicare system.

CASE STUDY I
Summarized

A middle-aged man suffers a mild heart attack and is hospitalized. Fortunately, the episode is uncomplicated. He spends 10 days recuperating in a hospital even though only five are medically necessary.

Retold

Bed Blocking — Because hospitals receive block grants, administrators have an incentive to fill beds with low-needs patients — they are cheaper to take care of and thus consume less of the global budget.

After five days, uncomplicated heart attack patients are essentially using only hotel-like services — inexpensive laundry and food services — rather than expensive medical services such as internist consultations, medications, and EKGs. Hospital administrators have an incentive to keep beds filled with this type of patient.

CASE STUDY 2
Summarized

An elderly woman suffers the aches and pains of old age. Her chief complaint is a minor back problem, which is controlled with aspirin. Yet she finds a doctor who runs countless tests on her, prescribes drugs, and sees her routinely. The follow-ups are unnecessary and unproductive, but the woman enjoys the attention.

Retold

The Patient as Overconsumer — A patient has a minor pain. She finds it inconvenient and sets out to cure it without consideration for cost — she isn't, after all, held financially accountable for her actions. When two physicians conclude that nothing more can be done, she decides to find another one. Why not? The visits cost her nothing. The new physician spends a great deal of money accomplishing little, but the patient enjoys the attention.

The Doctor as Overprovider — A young physician finds an easy source of money: an elderly patient with no serious conditions. The frequent visits are fast and effortless.

These mutually beneficial abuses of the system occur all the time. Occasionally, an extreme example will surface in the news. A few years back, the media reported the story of a woman who made 387 visits to doctors in one year (Priest, "Condition"). Such extremes are rare, but the mentality isn't.

CASE STUDY 3
Summarized

A young man under the strain of heavy academic pursuits suffers from headaches that are stress related. When he is offered a diagnostic test, he seizes the opportunity.

Retold

The MRI Scanner as High-Tech Counselling — The patient suffers from stress and has manifested physical signs. His doctor offers him an unnecessary and expensive test to confirm the diagnosis. From the patient's point of view, there's no need to contemplate such costs. The "safer rather than sorry" attitude prevails at a cost of hundreds of dollars.

4.8 Perverse Incentives and the Evolution of Medicare

Using the list in the previous section, we can summarize the major perverse incentives.

For the patient, there's the perverse incentive to overuse the system. Not directly responsible for the costs, a patient needn't think twice before using medical services. The incentive to consume for the sake of convenience and peace of mind is strong. As a joint government-medical association task force observed in 1977, demand becomes "infinite."

For the physician, there's the perverse incentive to overservice the patient. Paid by the service, many doctors instinctively provide too many services — they run more tests, provide more treatments, and do more follow-ups.

For the health care administrator, there's the perverse incentive to preserve and enhance the global budget. Granted a block allocation from the province, the hospital administrator must focus on the budget's bottom line rather than on the overall well-being of the health care system. Thus, practices such as bed blocking become common.

Why do these incentives exist? Simply put, because the medicare system has corrupted the basic doctor-patient relationship. By changing the nature of this relationship — by freeing patients from concerns about costs and by distorting the need for a physician to tend to patients first and foremost — medicare created malevolent incentives for both the providers and consumers of health care. The result: inefficient and wasteful health care at a high cost.

★ ★ ★

There's one more player in this game: the politician. In a publicly funded system, health care decisions are ultimately influenced by political considerations. Even before medicare, politicians involved themselves in many aspects of health care. For political benefit, governments across the country put up hospitals — too many of them. But after medicare was introduced, politicians soon found themselves in the less popular position of trying to control costs rather than simply spending money.

Medicare has evolved over the past three decades. Its history has been influenced by perverse incentives — and by the efforts of politicians to temper them.

The Golden Era

When medicare was introduced, politicians had little need to worry about costs. Canada's population was young and healthy. The economy was booming. The high-tech, high-cost revolution had yet to take place. Governments spent freely. In many ways, medicare was successful in its early days because it was untested. This first period was its golden era.

In debates over health care, people are often quick to point out that medicare once worked so well. They recall the golden era fondly as a time when hospitals were clean and new, when doctors were happy and ever helpful, when most Canadians rated the system as excellent. It was a time when many people proudly — and probably rightly — considered our health care system the best in the world.

But the problems that have grown to fruition today were nascent in this golden era. The root problem with medicare, after all, is structural, and it was during this time that the structure was established. The problems then, of course, were just seeds. Few analysts considered that, by making the system "free" to patients, the basic doctor-patient relationship would be corrupted. People didn't anticipate that the ready access to health services they enjoyed would one day be replaced by such lengthy waiting lists that a weekly newsmagazine could fill its front cover with pictures of patients who had suffered while waiting for treatment (see "Victims of Medicare"). People such as Justice Emmett Hall, whose royal commission report had established the framework for a national health care system, could gloat over their achievements, but the forces that would eventually result in an exodus of talented physicians, including Hall's own son, were already in place.

The Restricted-Supply Era

Predictably, the golden era didn't last long. It soon gave way to a harsher time in medicare's history, the restricted-supply era. Politicians soon discovered that Canadians were exceeding government capacity to finance the costs. Health care budgets continued to grow, but a decline in the quality of care was noticeable. For the first time, waiting lists emerged. During this era, they became so common that Canadians didn't even blink when a provincial minister of health said, "Waiting lists are not going to disappear in Canada. They're an accepted part of the system" (qtd. in Robert Walker, "Waiting Lists").

This development had much to do with two trends that continue to this day. The first trend was demographic: the program was introduced at a time when the Canadian population was young and healthy, with half under the age of 21. The median age of Canada's population was only 25 when Parliament passed the National Medical Insurance Act. In the subsequent years, the median age hit 30. Today the median age is approaching 40. An aging population means that new demands are placed on the health care system.

The second trend was the advance of medical technology. In areas such as diagnostic equipment and pharmaceuticals, major breakthroughs have taken place over the last three decades. And while the MRI scanners and channel blockers (antihypertensives) are capable of doing more than the X-ray machines and blood pressure medications of yesterday, they have dramatically increased the potential for funds to be spent on health services.

During the restricted-supply era, politicians were forced to look at ways of controlling health care costs. It was during this time that provincial governments turned out health care report after health care report. Despite the ideological differences between the governments, the approaches to dealing with the health care system were relatively similar. From right-leaning Alberta to left-leaning Nova Scotia, provincial governments decided to address the unchecked demand of consumers for health services by tempering the supply of these services. People could still see specialists without cost, but their ability to see them was reduced. Diagnostic tests were as free as the air, but governments were reluctant to buy the machines to perform these tests. "Reforms" universally restricted the supply of health services and included reductions in the number of medical graduates, restrictions in access to specialists, closures of hospital beds, deinsurance of certain services, restrictions in physician billing, limitations on high-tech equipment, and so on.

These changes, coupled with the increased demands of an aging population, meant that waiting lists developed. Although no provincial report mentioned rationing through waiting, it was (and is) the way in which provincial governments largely decided to curb excess demand. As in the old Soviet system, Canadians discovered that everything was free but nothing was readily available. So now they must line up. For tests. For surgery. For the basic health care they need.

No Canadian politician has ever mentioned the use of waiting lists, but they comprise the most powerful tool used to control costs. Politicians in other countries have been more candid. Enoch Powell, the former British minister of health, argued in his reflections on the National Health Service that waiting lists have served this role.

And while governments have quietly adopted this approach, its effects on quality care — its *human* costs — are rarely considered. As discussed in earlier chapters, waiting lists are a cruel way to ration health care. People on the lists often wait in pain, some grow sicker, and many become anxious.

The Central-Management Era

In the past few years, Canada has embarked on a new era in medicare, the central-management era. Frustrated by redundancies and inefficiencies within the system, provincial governments have opted to try to manage it, and they now involve themselves in practically every aspect of health care delivery.

The shift in thinking was well summarized in a 26 April 1996 speech given by Jim Wilson, then the minister of health in Ontario. He explained how he planned to transform the ministry: "We will go from being simply a passive payer to an active manager." This approach symbolizes the new thinking: improvements in health care delivery require direct government control.

Consider, for example, the reforms of the Manitoba government. Since taking office in 1988, Premier Gary Filmon has privatized crown corporations and introduced tough balanced-budget legislation. The Tories are now contemplating a broadly based tax cut. Conservative critics argue that more could be done, but there's no doubt that Filmon isn't a believer in big government.

Yet, when it comes to the health portfolio, his philosophy is very different. In early 1998, Conservatives created a powerful superboard to run the nine Winnipeg hospitals, thereby leaving the institutions' boards virtually impotent. They introduced a similar reform for the rural hospitals. In January, the minister of health announced that Manitoba Health would take over all diagnostic testing. The reforms, then, have focused on big government running the medicare system.

What would drive Filmon, a moderate fiscal conservative with a dislike of large government, to such measures? Try a hospital system that lacks even the most basic computer tracking of patients — many tests are often duplicated because different departments don't have access to the same information. A system in which the waiting period for an important diagnostic test such as a bone scan can be reduced from two years to four months by simple political pressure. A system in which the nine urban hospitals routinely run deficits because of the "unreasonable" fiscal restraint of the government but still manage to spend over $2.5 million subsidizing cafeteria food.

Provincial governments, like Manitoba's, see these sorts of problems and come to a simple conclusion: government management is better than no management. In a small way, they're right — a one-pack-a-day smoking habit seems like a real improvement compared with a two-packs-a-day habit.

The provincial reform efforts — greater government management and restricted supply of services — have attempted to offset the perverse incentives within the medicare system. Some efforts have worked well, others haven't. Rather than trying to force patients not to overconsume or to force doctors not to overservice, it makes more sense to replace the perverse incentives with common sense. After all, an efficient system doesn't try to change people; it only attempts to work within the confines of human nature.

There is, however, a more dangerous aspect to the reforms.

4.9 Anatomy of a Crisis

It is ironic that Mrs. Jeannine Lacombe received so much attention after her death. Suffering from chest pain, the Montrealer went to the nearest hospital emergency room in February 1998. Four hours later, a physician finally looked at the 66-year-old woman who lay on a stretcher in the hallway. She was dead.

On that early February morning, Maisonneuve-Rosemont Hospital was crowded with 63 patients in a ward designed to accommodate a maximum of 34. Only 3 of Montreal's 24 emergency rooms weren't overflowing with double or triple their capacities.

And the problem wasn't confined to Montreal.[8] In Toronto, a five-year-old boy died in an ER five hours after arriving. He, too, never saw a physician. At times that February, the situation was so bad that nurses fought with ambulance attendants over the stretchers patients were brought in on — having so few beds available, the hospital staff needed every stretcher they could get or patients would have had to lie on the floor. The assistant director of operations for Toronto Ambulance commented that the hospitals were refusing ambulance patients more often and for longer periods than at any time in the previous 27 years (Gratzer, "Guest Column").

In Winnipeg, the hospitals had routinely been on "redirect" — meaning that they only accept patients needing critical care; all others have to go elsewhere — and "critical care bypass" — indicating that they are too crowded to receive even critical patients. During an eight-hour period in mid-February, all urban hospitals went on critical care bypass. A local doctor joked, "It's pretty simple. Just don't have a heart attack in Winnipeg." Some elderly patients waited up to five days in hospital corridors before being admitted to a bed. At least they had company — a total of 107 patients were waiting in hallways at one point.

In Calgary, a physician discovered that overcrowding was so bad in the emergency room of the Rocky View Hospital that when he arrived for work patients were standing in front of the glass doors — in the parking lot. The ER and the foyer were already full. "I have never seen anything like that in all the years I have been practising." The Regional Health Authority, responding to the overcrowding, openly contemplated cancelling all elective surgeries. By month's end, health officials in Edmonton had done so.

Dozens of other stories could be told from that February period. From coast to coast, newspapers reported similar problems. With emergency rooms filled to capacity, patients were routinely left for days on gurneys in hallways; elective procedures were cancelled; and patients waited for hours, sometimes days, to receive proper medical attention.

The frustration felt by physicians was palpable. Consider the following description by a Hamilton emergency physician:

The emergency department in which I work has 21 beds. As I write this, 17 of those beds are occupied by patients who need to be admitted to hospital but for whom no ward bed is available. Two beds are filled with patients currently being investigated by the emergency room physician. They likely will also need admission to non-existent hospital beds.

Thus, I am starting my day with a department that has only two beds accessible to the public. This is before most of my patients arrive. My consolation is that yesterday was worse. (Kollek)

In many ways, the health care system collapsed for a four-week period. What happened? Some analysts dismiss the significance of these reports, arguing that a combination of winter storms and the flu placed an unusual strain on the system. These two factors certainly contributed to the level of overcrowding, but they aren't in themselves adequate explanations. Northern US states, such as North Dakota and Michigan, would have been just as affected by winter storms and the flu, yet emergency room overcrowding remained a Canadian crisis.

A more satisfying if startling explanation is that medicare has slowly eroded to the point where even minor stresses can wreak havoc. Provincial governments, in their efforts to achieve "cost containment," have embarked on a series of "reforms" with little thought given to the real consequences. Patients are discharged earlier from hospitals, often too early. Others wait for treatment, some developing complications. Hospital beds are closed, reducing the ability of doctors to admit patients. All these factors played a role in the ER crisis of February 1998. To make matters worse, government bureaucrats have developed elaborate controls on spending, reducing the ability of the system to react quickly to fluctuating needs.

The situation in February 1998 was foreseeable. It was. Hospital emergency rooms have been getting more and more busy — and overcrowded. According to Capital Health Authority figures, Edmonton had 489 red-alert hours (when hospitals can divert all but critical cases) from July to September 1996. Over the same quarter in 1997, the red-alert hours hit 796, a 63% increase. In a year, the average wait in Edmonton emergency rooms grew from 7.5 hours to 9.3 hours (Sillars 12). And the emergency wards in Montreal were filled to 155% capacity in February 1996, a year before Mrs. Lacombe died in such a ward while waiting for treatment ("Emergency").

So, a decade after health care reform had become the urgent impulse of every province, Canadians were faced with a health care system so rigid as to collapse under the strain of a flu and a couple of freak storms.

Is there likely to be such a disaster in the future? Will February be known in cities such as Calgary, Montreal, and Halifax as the month of emergency room crowding, the way April is associated with spring and October with snow? As noted in the introduction to this book, similar problems occurred in 1999. And those emergency room crises are symptoms of a larger problem. As long as provincial governments seek Band-Aid solutions for the problems of the health care system — as long as they embrace miracle solutions such as bed closures and regional health boards — similar episodes will recur.

5

Demographics, Drugs, and Disaster

Boom, Bust, and Echo: *How to Profit from the Coming Demographic Shift* is a major publishing success, having sold more than a quarter of a million copies and staying on the best-seller list for over 100 weeks. Written by a bespectacled economics professor from the University of Toronto with the help of an accomplished journalist, it describes the aging of the Canadian population — and how to profit from it. Using demographic analysis, the authors offer predictions on everything from housing prices to crime rates.

Part of the attraction of the book — besides the obvious financial pull — is the absolute confidence with which the authors write. Dr. David Foot and Daniel Stoffman understand the effects of our demographic shifts on education, leisure activities, and education. They don't speculate why tennis was popular in the mid-1980s but not a decade later; rather, they know that this shift was "inevitable" (1). Demographics aren't merely factors in people's behaviour; indeed, "demographics explain about two-thirds of everything" (2).

Boom, Bust, and Echo may be brash, but it is one of the most important books written in Canada this decade, for Foot and Stoffman understand what so few politicians are able to grasp:

> Demography, the study of human populations, is the most powerful — and underutilized — tool we have to understand the past and to foretell the future. Demographics affect every one of us as individuals, far more than most of us have ever imagined. They also play a pivotal role in the economic and social life of our country. (2)

The shifting demographics that they recognize and detail are useful because they have enormous impact on public policy.

5.1 Getting Older

The popularity of *Boom, Bust, and Echo* and the discussions it has sparked indicate that Canadians are increasingly aware of the shifting demographics. In a nutshell, we know that our society is getting older.

And when it comes to public policy, experts and politicians are increasingly willing to discuss the effects of this shift on the Canada Pension Plan (CPP). Those with a statist bias have argued that the way to increase the long-term sustainability of the plan is to increase contributions, thereby enlarging the pot of money available to retirees. Those with an individualist slant have argued for a form of privatization modelled on the reforms of countries such as Chile. In 1997, the federal government announced its vision for reforming the CPP: substantially hiked contributions. Critics of this approach — the C.D. Howe Institute, the Canadian Taxpayers Federation, and the Reform Party of Canada, to name a few — have offered detailed alternative plans.

Ironically, as much as politicians and experts are willing to acknowledge the demographic problem with our pensions and offer different visions of reform, practically nothing is said about the future of health care. Medicare, after all, suffers from the same basic demographic problem as the CPP. Today's workers are paying for today's medicare users, but what happens when there are many more users and relatively fewer taxpayers? Yet the C.D. Howe Institute and the Canadian Taxpayers Federation have not released a plan on "saving" medicare. The Reform Party's position on medicare has changed dramatically over the years, but it has never attempted to address the sustainability of health care.

Or consider John Richards's *Retooling the Welfare State: What's Right, What's Wrong, What's to Be Done.* The author, a former NDP MLA from Saskatchewan, offers a scathing (and brilliant) critique of the welfare state. When it comes to the CPP, he recognizes the demographics and suggests that, while reform is needed, Chilean-style individual accounts are preferable to the federal government's strategy. But when medicare comes up, criticisms and positive suggestions end: "Canada's health care system is clearly a part of its welfare state that works" (130). Indeed, there's no mention of any demographic problem in the entire chapter dedicated to medicare (see 118–32).

This oversight may seem trivial, but it isn't. Sustainability is the most significant health care issue in this country — more important to the future of medicare than hospital closures, physician compensation, or any of the other issues politicians and experts are willing to discuss. As Philander Chase Johnson wrote in *Everybody's Magazine*, "Cheer up, the worst is yet to come." Written decades before medicare was even a sparkle in the eye of Tommy Douglas, the words perfectly reflect the outlook for the system — the problems with medicare are only going to get worse with time. We can go further: the odds are, unless significant changes are made, medicare will go bankrupt.

Bankruptcy may seem like a harsh prediction. It isn't. We can justify this claim in one sentence: the use of medical services is strongly influenced by age — the older we are, the more often we need to use the health care system.

In *Boom, Bust, and Echo*, Foot and Stoffman provide the stats to illustrate the point:

> Reliance on doctors increases in a person's 40s, but above-average use of hospitals doesn't occur until the mid-50s. Then it takes off. By the time you are in your late 70s, you will use hospitals five times more than your lifetime average rate of use. If you survive until your late 80s, you will use hospitals 12 times more than your lifetime average. As for doctors, by your late 70s you will call on them twice as much as your lifetime average, and in your 80s, 2.5 times as much. (165)

Others have reported similar findings. A recent study on health care utilization, for example, found that the 65–74 age group uses approximately two and a half times the number of services as the 15–44 age group (Globerman and Vining 17). Statistics Canada reports that out of every dollar spent on health in Canada today, 39¢ is spent on the 65+ group. Another 20¢ is spent by the 45–65 group. In other words, 59¢ of every dollar spent on health care is for those in their middle age or senior years (Baxter and Rambo 1).

These stats make sense. After all, a 70-year-old man is much more likely to require treatment for cancer or heart disease than, say, a teenager. Additionally, older citizens often require more costly treatments involving hospitalization and long-term facilities. Geriatric diseases (Alzheimer's, Parkinson's, and so on) are expensive.

Unfortunately, demographers predict that Canada's population is getting older, primarily because of the baby boom generation. Postwar children number about 9.8 million, or a third of the population. In 1997, the oldest members of this group started turning 50 (Foot and

Stoffman 163). With this important birthday, the largest single cohort in Canada will be not only paying for part of the costs of medicare but also, in increasing numbers, utilizing the program. As comedian Billy Crystal observed in *City Slickers*, the fifties are the age of elective surgery.

And as baby boomers get even older, a more dramatic shift will occur. Around 2012, they will start retiring. Within the two decades thereafter, a large group in the population will be utilizing health care but will no longer be contributing to the tax base. The implication is clear: if money is tight now, it will get much tighter later.

The Office of the Superintendent of Financial Services attempted to calculate the tax rates needed to pay for the medicare system in the coming years, taking into account only the shifting demographics (Clemens and Ramsay 7). The results are anything but encouraging. In 1995, the average family paid a tax rate of 48%. In 2010, the average family's taxes will need to jump to 58.5%. And increases continue to 74.5% in 2025 and then 94.5% in 2040.

When the majority of baby boomers are in their senior years, medicare at today's costs would require tax rates at the absurd level of 94.5% The study's findings are even more discouraging when the assumptions are analysed — the estimates are based on a fairly rosy economic outlook. The projection, for instance, assumes that wages will grow by 4.5% a year.

The Urban Futures Institute, based in British Columbia, projects that real health expenditures will grow by 80% over the next 40 years. The estimates are based on the assumption that, over those four decades, the number of people 45 or older will grow as a portion of the population from one-third to one-half (Clemens and Ramsay 2).

5.2 The Cost of Progress

But if the projections seem bad, the reality could be worse. The Urban Futures Institute, for instance, only looked at shifting demographics in its analysis. But health costs aren't just influenced by the age of the population. Previous spending patterns illustrate the point. Between 1980 and 1994, health expenditures rose from $22.4 billion to $72.5 billion — an increase of 224%. Some of this phenomenal rise can be explained by inflation. A 1994 dollar isn't worth as much as a 1980 dollar. But if we account for inflation, demographics aren't enough to completely explain the rise. Of every dollar more spent on health care, 8.4¢ can be chalked up to Canada's aging population. Almost four times that amount — a full 30.4¢ of the new health care dollar — can be pinned on increased health spending (2–3).

Why did governments spend so much more on health care at the end of this 15-year period? Simply put, because they could. The possibilities for spending money on health care are growing by leaps and bounds as the face of medical care is transformed by unprecedented advances. Every aspect of medicine — surgical treatment, pharmaceuticals, diagnostic testing — is affected by the "high-tech, high-cost" medical revolution.

Projections of health care costs in the future fail to take into account the long-term consequences of this revolution. The Urban Futures Institute naïvely assumes that in 2035 patients will want 1990s-style medicine. Would we be content today with the medicine of 40 years ago? Would we be happy in a health care system today in which bypass surgery is unheard of and diagnostic equipment such as MRI and CT scanners don't exist?

It's difficult to judge what medicine will look like in the future. If recent history is any indication, future possibilities for health care will be awesome. Consider the major advances of the last three decades. Dr. Caroline Poplin lists them in an article for the *Wilson Quarterly*:

> The results came in a rush: widespread use of ventilators, the development of intensive care units, and the computer-assisted tomography (CT) scanner, the introduction of cardiac bypass surgery, all in the 1970s; fiber-optic devices and magnetic resonance imagers (MRIs) in the 1980s, which made possible diagnoses that heretofore had required invasive surgery, along with recombinant DNA pharmaceuticals, and materials and techniques for total joint replacement; and, finally, in the 1990s, laparascopic surgeries, which permit surgeons to perform major procedures such as gall bladder removal and chest lymph-node biopsy through a few inch-long slits, thus allowing the patient to go home the same day. (15)

It's difficult to fully appreciate how much modern medicine has improved our lives. These advances have improved not only healing — doctors have a greater ability to diagnose and treat disease — but also quality of life. A hip replacement, after all, doesn't save a life, but the mobility it grants the patient is impressive. An elderly woman, for example, will no longer be confined to her apartment; she will be free to pursue her daily activities.

The catch is that each advance in medicine comes with a price tag. Consider the following scenario. A young man falls from his bicycle and bumps his head. At the turn of the century, a family physician could only perform a handful of superficial neurological tests on a patient suffering from head trauma. He could have tested the patient's reflexes — the Babinski sign, eye dilation, and stretch response — and looked for deficits in the basic functions. Can the patient hear in both ears? Can he see with both eyes? Most of the tests would have required little more than a bright light, a blunt instrument, and some time. Today a doctor in a similar situation would not only be able to perform these crude tests but would also have a virtual arsenal of high-tech diagnostic weapons available to determine the type and extent of the head injury: the CT scan, the MRI, and the EEG, to name a few. But these tests come at high costs. An MRI scanner costs millions of dollars, and each scan costs $850. As new technologies develop, the possibilities — and the costs associated with them — continue to increase.

There's a final problem to note about the future of health care in Canada: the infrastructure is getting old. Many hospitals were built in the 1960s. Basic machinery — X-rays and the like — is also aging.

It's difficult to judge the deterioration of our health care infrastructure. Provincial governments have been reluctant to replace aging equipment, opting instead for the cheaper (and short-term) goal of maintaining existing machinery. When asked about the condition of the diagnostic equipment in hospitals, a radiologist in Alberta replied with exasperation: "it seems the government is content to hold things together with chicken wire and Band-Aids." The doctor partly blamed the problem on the bureaucratic process needed to purchase new equipment. "In my office, if we want new equipment, I contact four different contractors. I get the best price and order. It takes about two months. For a hospital to do the same, it takes about two years."

Bureaucratic problems aside, the lack of attention to capital infrastructure has dark consequences for the future. It's possible today to spend less on health care because of the tremendous investments in infrastructure in the past — hospital reconstruction isn't immediately necessary because many buildings were put up in the 1960s and 1970s. But chicken wire and Band-Aids only work for so long. In a decade or two — when baby boomers start heavily using the health care system — the infrastructure will be old and decaying. The low-cost maintenance that most facilities perform won't be sufficient. Indeed, the type of capital upgrading required will be widespread and costly. Entire hospitals will require rebuilding. Likewise, X-ray machines and other diagnostic equipment may be adequate today, but in a decade or two they will need to be replaced.

5.3 The Tip of the Iceberg

"We are seeing now only the tip of the iceberg," observed Stephen Harper, the president of the National Citizens' Coalition, in conversation. His point is that advancing technology coupled with an aging population means the worst is yet to come.

But such a view sharply contradicts views expressed publicly by experts. Consider the comments made by Stephen Lewis on *The National* on 4 February 1997. Lewis, the CEO of Saskatchewan's Health Services Utilization and Research Commission, stated that medicare was "in a time of transition." His point was simple: there may be problems with medicare today, but fear not, for tomorrow will be better. Lewis was trying to allay the growing concerns of Canadians about the state of the health care system. The concerns are hardly surprising — it's almost daily that we read news reports about medicare's problems.

But, as Lewis explained, worry is unnecessary. Transition, after all, suggests something that is temporary. And, after this period of transition, he implied, everything in health care would return to normal. As soothing and tempting as this message may be, it is hopelessly misleading. All the demographic evidence suggests that medicare is not in some brief period of change but in a long period of decline.

If patients are troubled today by lengthy waiting lists, overcrowded emergency rooms, and lackadaisical hospital standards, what will medicare be like in the coming years? Over the next 40 years, the number of seniors will double to a quarter of the total population. Such a demographic shift will create unprecedented stresses on the system. Waiting lists will continue to grow, emergency rooms will be seriously and regularly overcrowded, and the discontent of health care workers will escalate. This is not a transition. This is a transformation.

Lewis, however, isn't one man with one off-the-wall opinion. His view is shared by most of the prominent health care experts. Indeed, when he was interviewed on *The National*, he was asked to comment on the report of the National Forum on Health, which (as noted above) declared medicare "fundamentally sound." It's difficult to understand how the committee arrived at such a conclusion when the system is so riddled with perverse incentives.

Medicare is not fundamentally sound. It is, rather, *fundamentally unsound* in terms of its basic structure and in light of Canada's aging population.

6

Back to Basics

W HEN IT COMES to medicare, many consider Michael Decter a guru of sorts. A former deputy minister of health in Ontario — described on the back cover of his book by columnist Jeffrey Simpson as "one of the best and brightest public servants of his generation" — Decter is now a health care consultant and chair of the Canadian Institute for Health Information. He is frequently quoted by the *Globe and Mail* and other newspapers. And it's difficult to find a stronger proponent of medicare than Decter.

His book on the system, *Healing Medicare: Managing Health System Change the Canadian Way*, opens thus: "Medicare is among the most cherished of Canadian achievements." It is "a true Canadian success story" and "a national achievement" — all this in just the first paragraph (9). The preservation of medicare, writes Decter, is "the struggle"; these are fighting words, and no wonder — "To abandon the struggle would be to abandon our values. We will succeed" (254).

Decter recognizes, however, that medicare must be changed: *"It isn't reform that will bring about the demise of medicare but the absence of it"* (15). He sees himself as a champion not only of medicare but also of reform. So he identifies many problems with the system and then suggests possible reforms. The recommendations, however, are of limited imagination and practicality. Decter recognizes the misuse of medical services by patients and can only suggest tempering demand with "nurse call lines, video cassettes for patient education, and advertising campaigns to convince cold sufferers to visit a pharmacy not a doctor or a hospital" (179). He sees hospital mismanagement and recommends that hospital administrators "Ask the people who work there, all of them," as part of his "radical" plan to achieve efficiency (44). He notes the strength of rigid public sector unions and suggests that "bargaining agents need to overhaul . . . [their attitudes] toward the process and management as well" (103).

Decter should be praised for seeing medicare's woes.[1] Nonetheless,

his package of reforms is hopelessly inadequate. Patients misuse medical services because they have an incentive to do so in a "free" system,
and an advertising campaign is unlikely to change this behaviour.
Hospitals are mismanaged because block grants create little incentive for
them to be managed well, and employee surveys won't change attitudes.
Public sector unions can afford to take hard stands because their strikes
disrupt the entire system of health care, and promoting labour open-
mindedness amounts to wishful thinking.

Decter, in short, says practically nothing of value about reforms. His
ideas amount to tinkering. Why is this? Decter, after all, is acutely familiar with the system, having spent years in the civil service. But starting from the position that the foundation of medicare is beyond
question, he can't say much of value. And he is unwilling to admit that
his bias dooms his vision of change to a wish list.

Significantly, Decter sees the symptoms but not their underlying
causes. However, that he and other strong supporters of the system
acknowledge these shortcomings and, more importantly, the unsustain-
ability of the status quo marks a major turning point in the debate over
medicare.

Although Decter's solutions are unworkable, the alternatives are difficult to envision. The general acknowledgement that our health care
system needs to change is cause for celebration, but what's the next
step?

6.1 Medicare's Problems

Health care is a big problem — or, more correctly, several big problems.

First, health care is a *societal* problem. Canadians are getting older.
Over the next 40 years, the percentage of people over 65 will double to
a quarter of Canada's population. More seniors need more medical services. The wear and tear on hips and knees over the years destroys
these joints and reduce a person's mobility. Cataracts frequently form
as eyes age, thus limiting vision. Western eating habits take their toll
on coronary arteries and cause heart disease. These problems demand
expensive medical solutions: joint replacements, cataract surgeries, and
heart bypasses. The list of diseases common to an elderly population —
cancer, Alzheimer's, depression — stretches. Consider that the Canadian
Cancer Society forecasts a 70% increase in cancer diagnoses by 2010
based on the demographic trend (see National Cancer Institute of

Canada 23–38). And medical needs mean not simply life-saving measures but also home care, nursing homes, and other services to assist a person when age and disease limit independent living.

Second, health care is a *budgetary* problem. Health expenditures as a percentage of GDP stood at 6.1% in 1961. By the end of the 1990s, the percentage will probably exceed 10% — despite Canada's dramatic growth in wealth. Health care is the largest single expenditure in every province. Overall, the state spends in excess of $50 billion a year on health care. An aging population coupled with advances in medical technology promises to create unprecedented demands on government budgets.

Third, health care is an *economic* problem. Accounting for about a tenth of our national production, the health care sector is an integral part of the economy. Medicare, however, corrupts efficiency with its perverse incentives. With taxpayers spending roughly 21¢ on every dollar earned, this inefficiency means that less money is available for Canadians to spend in other ways — or to save.

Fourth, health care is a *political* problem. While politicians may prefer to change the subject or to speak in platitudes, polls show that health care ranks as one of the highest concerns for Canadians. Moreover, they are growing pessimistic about the future of medicare.

Fifth, health care is a *moral* problem. As waiting lists continue to grow, Canadians must increasingly wonder why more and more people are forced to suffer both emotional and physical pain. In one of the wealthiest countries on Earth, it is unacceptable that this situation be allowed to continue.

These are big problems. These are urgent problems. These are complicated problems. What now? Reinventing the health care system is no simple task. Even though the impetus for change is great, the health care system involves billions of dollars and hundreds of thousands of doctors, nurses, and support staff.

The type of reform needed requires changes to almost every aspect of health care delivery in Canada. Consider the following basic questions that need to be answered.

- Should we close hospitals to save money? If so, which hospitals? Should we close redundant wards? If so, which wards?
- Should we attempt to centralize hospital purchasing? How would we coordinate this?

- Should chronic abusers of the system be punished? If so, how?
- Should we introduce new regulations to reduce abuse? How comprehensive should these regulations be? Would we create too much red tape with such an effort?
- To save money, should we stop funding certain procedures and pharmaceuticals that aren't medically essential? How do we determine what is medically essential and what isn't?
- Do we have too many physicians? How do we determine if we do? And, if we can, how do we reduce their numbers? What about nurses and support staff?

Hospital management, chronic abuse, procedural funding, staffing — the list of issues is depressingly long. The process of answering them and effecting real change is daunting. Redesigning health care delivery requires the collection of tremendous amounts of data. Union contracts need to be renegotiated. Staff must be relocated. Hospitals need to be shut down. All this — but would these changes even work?

There's no guarantee that cost-saving changes to primary care delivery won't result in greater (and more costly) hospital utilization. Or that changes to physician billing won't reduce the work ethic. Or that hospital-funding changes to address the perverse incentives won't merely replace them with a new set of perverse incentives. Worst of all, some of the questions may not even be answerable. How many hospital beds are needed per 1,000 people?

Even if such questions can be answered, who can make such decisions without being affected by his or her own biases? Should doctors and nurses be trusted to make the right decisions? Disinterested third parties may be the natural choice, but they lack the expertise. And if we can agree on the right answers from the right people, can the necessary changes really be made? Health care, after all, involves hundreds of thousands of workers, many unionized, all stakeholders.

Perhaps the problem is that, while the questions may be valid, the basic assumption is incorrect. Is it the government's role to run the health care system? From this statist perspective, reforming the system is about micromanaging health care better. Hence, questions such as "How many hospitals should there be?" seem relevant. There is, of course, an alternative: cut the Gordian knot rather than trying to unravel it one thread at a time.

The question of how to reform the health care system is complex and controversial. Deciding how to get there is more difficult than deciding exactly where "there" is. Let's take a step backward and ask a much simpler question. *What type of health care system do we want?*

6.2 The Five Pillars of Health Care

Canadians demand certain basic characteristics in a health care system. People speak of the five principles of the Canada Health Act, but the obsession with these principles misses the point. Provincial portability, for example, may be nice, but it isn't as essential as timeliness of care. Portability between provinces is a regulatory agreement worth pursuing, but no one will die if portability is not enshrined in federal law but left to the provinces to negotiate between themselves.

The defining characteristics of a health care system should speak to the basic pillars upon which good health care rests. Following are the *five pillars* of health care.

1. *Quality.* Canadians need a system that provides quality medical care. The latest technology should be used to diagnose and treat citizens; medical facilities should be modern and well equipped; physicians, nurses, and other providers must be highly trained and skilled.
2. *Timeliness.* Illness should be diagnosed and treated quickly. Doing so makes economic sense — long waits mean people are less productive. And timeliness is morally necessary, for forcing patients to wait in pain for treatment is cruel and wrong.
3. *Cost effectiveness.* The system needs to produce acceptable results for the funds put into it. Wasting precious resources on, say, unnecessary procedures and unproductive administrators isn't worthwhile.
4. *Patient orientation.* The health care system must serve the patients, not the providers. Additionally, patients — not bureaucrats — must be the ultimate decision makers about their individual care. The choice of physicians and treatments must rest with the patient.
5. *Accessibility.* Regardless of financial circumstances, no Canadian should be deprived of the opportunity to get the medical care he or she requires.

These five pillars are hardly controversial. Could even the strongest of medicare proponents suggest that timeliness isn't important? Would any advocate of two-tiered health care doubt that quality is essential? But it's alarming to realize the extent to which the present system fails. On nearly each characteristic above, medicare falls short.

Quality

With limited investments in capital expenditures such as building reno-
vations and technologically advanced equipment, the quality of care
has suffered.

Consider, for example, a straightforward arthroscopic surgery on
the shoulder described recently in a medical journal (see Jones 297).
The older equipment requires an incision of 15 cm. This incision affects
recovery time: the patient will miss four months of work. With state-
of-the-art equipment (not available in the medicare system), the same
surgery requires only a tiny incision — and a six-week recovery time. In
both cases, the shoulder heals, but there's a clear difference in the quality
of care.

Diagnostic testing equipment, such as MRI scanners, isn't readily
available except under extreme circumstances. As a result, doctors are
forced to make do with older, and thus more limiting, equipment.

The exodus of Canada's best and brightest physicians has further
hurt quality.

Timeliness

Timeliness doesn't simply mean that emergency care is readily available. It also means the ability of the health care system to promptly
diagnose and treat illnesses. Of course, no health care system is without delays, but there's a profound difference between a heart bypass
surgery being scheduled within a week or within a year.

As discussed above, waiting lists plague Canada's system of health
care delivery. A reasonable estimate is that well over 100,000 Canadians
are waiting for some form of health care — many are in pain, and
some will die.

Waiting lists aren't growing pains — that is, a problem that medicare
will one day move beyond as it matures. Rather, such lists are an important way of tempering the excessive demand in our "free" health care
system.

Patient Orientation

With the state as payer, patient orientation diminishes. For one thing,
the doctor-state relationship replaces the doctor-patient relationship.

To bill successfully, physicians are forced to meet not their patients' needs but the regulations of the state.

In fact, the influence of the state extends to nearly every aspect of health care delivery. Certain drugs, for instance, may be of proven benefit but aren't readily available due to their high costs. The use of Streptokinase, a less effective post-heart attack medication, as opposed to tPA is a case in point.

And the state as payer means that an artificial system of funding is created. Block funding to institutional providers (e.g., hospitals), for instance, means that they have little incentive to concern themselves with the communities they serve.

Cost Effectiveness

Is Canada getting good value for the billions of taxpayers' dollars invested in medicare? With limited accounting practices and tracking of patient outcomes, it's impossible to determine the cost effectiveness of medicare. Nevertheless, it seems evident that medicare isn't well organized.

Corruption of the doctor-patient relationship invites misuse of the system. Patients overconsume health services, and doctors overprovide these services. The bills add up. And the funding of institutional providers, allowing hospitals to function as a cartel, is certainly ineffective.

There are many examples to support this argument. Consider the waiting lists for bone scans in Manitoba. In 1997, the newly appointed minister of health decided to reduce the waiting times for bone scans — patients were waiting nearly two years for the basic diagnostic test. To clear the backlog, St. Boniface Hospital, which performed the testing for the province, requested a new machine and the hiring of several new employees — at an overall cost of $400,000. When the minister investigated the situation, he discovered that the present machine was utilized only two days a week. The waiting list was cleared in three months, at a cost of only $40,000. A Quebec government study found that costs for delivering standard procedures varied between hospitals by as much as 50%.

Accessibility

For financial accessibility, medicare seems to deserve a passing grade. Generally, Canadians are able to access the health care system without concern for cost. The deinsurance of certain services and the introduction of limited user fees worry some because of their potential to threaten accessibility. For the most part, however, these concerns are unfounded.

But to say that our health care system is "accessible" amounts to an equivocation of sorts. Financial circumstances, after all, won't keep an individual from getting the MRI scan he or she needs — waiting lists and government guidelines will. Yes, Canadians can marvel at the accessibility of medicare, but the question remains: "What do we have access to?" Dr. Gabor Lantos answers this question about access with examples from his own practice: "a patient with liver failure who never had an 'elective' admission and whose spouse had to stay home from work to provide care, an elderly patient with acute renal failure who was never offered dialysis, and two patients needing spine operations who waited months for MRI scans."

It's remarkable that when medicare is held to the light — that is, tested against basic and uncontroversial criteria of quality, timeliness, cost effectiveness, consumer orientation, and accessibility — the system fails so miserably. A shock, in many ways, because Canadians are used to hearing endless praise for medicare. It is supposed to be "the best health care system in the world," yet tens of thousands wait for treatment, many of them in pain. Medicare is "what makes us Canadian," but up-to-date equipment isn't available, so many doctors today are forced to practise decade-old medicine or worse.

Nearly none of these pointed criticisms comes from Canada's health care analysts and health economists — those who study the field for a living and should bring such issues to light are silent. These so-called experts are hopelessly biased. They don't see medicare as a means to an end: solid health care for Canadians. Instead, it has become an end in itself. It is, in their view, more than a social program — it's a struggle for the soul of the country.

Thus, proponents of medicare have tried to frame the debate about medicare and its alternatives as a struggle between a perfect system (the envy of the world) and who knows what. Phrased this way, medicare always looks good. But the debate for Canada isn't between perfection and risky alternatives. Medicare is a mediocre system, and it will only get worse with time. The debate over medicare is between a system doomed to failure and alternatives that could potentially provide excellence and affordability.

Given what's at stake, it's not surprising to hear the endless slogan-eering. Proponents of the system attack all new ideas as an "American-ization" of our health care system, vilify opponents by questioning their patriotism, and become fearmongers by suggesting that even the most modest changes to medicare will result in health being available only to the rich.

These attacks are born not of strength but of weakness. Medicare is getting harder and harder to defend.

*　*　*

These five characteristics are vital, for they define excellence in health care. No one would debate that excellence in health care is an impor-tant goal. Health care, after all, is a basic need. Without it, both the quality and the quantity of life are diminished.

But health care isn't the only need. Basic needs also include food, shelter, and clothing. In this list, in fact, health care is in some ways the least important need. Without proper clothing and shelter, it is difficult to live in almost any Canadian city during the brisk winter. And how long can a person survive without food? Such arguments, of course, are intellectually interesting but not of much practical value — each one of these needs is important.

Applying the five pillars to the other basic needs, we will likely find the results curious. Consumer orientation: when looking for a jacket at The Bay, do you believe that the store is trying to serve your needs — that is, provide you with a jacket you want that fits your body — or the needs of the clothing companies — a one-size-fits-all jacket that is the cheapest to manufacture and distribute? Timeliness: how many times have you been homeless waiting for any apartment to become avail-able? The answers are fairly clear.

Let's consider our food system in a little more detail. *Quality*: we can purchase an incredible variety of quality food, from the exotic cuisine of foreign lands to the wholesome goodness of locally grown flour. *Timeliness*: food is always readily available, even in the wee hours of the morning. *Cost effectiveness*: most restaurants and grocery stores are cost effective; if not, they go bankrupt. *Consumer orientation*: food is pro-duced to be sold, so producers have a strong incentive to meet the needs and desires of consumers. *Accessibility*: all Canadians have access to basic foods. True, not everyone can afford caviar and lox, but no one starves.

In fact, of the four basic needs, health care is the only one that fails to meet the five characteristics. What distinguishes it from the others? Health care delivery is burdened with excessive regulations and controls, competition is scarce, and both providers and users see no connection between their choices and the costs associated with them.

This isn't to suggest that the government has no role to play in, say, the food system. Government plays the role of watchdog, ensuring food quality through inspections and standards. Government also plays the role of consumer advocate, requiring companies to disclose the contents and the nutritional value of their products. And government plays the role of societal charity, redistributing income so that the poor are able to buy food.

The government, however, doesn't play the role of food purchaser, determining how many loafs of bread and slices of salami a community requires to satisfy its lunch needs; or the role of food planner, closing and amalgamating grocery stores to accommodate population shifts and to achieve cost savings; or the role of food manager, determining the wages of grocers and the budgets of grocery stores.

Such a comparison may seem profoundly unsatisfying: most people consider food products commonplace and modern medical care fascinating. Is a loaf of bread to be likened to an MRI scanner? Frozen chicken to a CT scan?

To illustrate the complexity of human interactions, economics professors often ask a simple question: "Who makes a pencil?" No one person, of course, actually makes a pencil. The wood, the paint, the eraser, the graphite, the metal band — these elements come from hundreds of companies in dozens of countries. Although the end product is common and inexpensive, the process involves the coordination of thousands of people (Friedman 18).

Likewise, bread may seem like a simple product, but it involves the efforts of many workers. The production of food is no less complicated than that of health care. The difference is the level of government intervention. With food delivery, government tempers the market. With health care, government has corrupted the market.

Consider that, in a normal market, problems are solved by consumers and producers pursuing their own self-interests.[2] Consumers tend to avoid waste and inefficiency because they usually result in higher prices. Instead, consumers seek good products at attractive prices offered by efficient suppliers. Producers search for less costly ways of delivering wanted goods — they reduce inefficiencies and develop innovative approaches. Pursuit of self-interest by consumers rewards efficient producers, and pursuit of self-interest by producers rewards cost-conscious consumers.

But these normal market processes — based on productive self-interest, if you will — have been replaced for health care by bureaucratic institutions, and normal market incentives have been replaced by bureaucratic rule making.

- In a normal marketplace, people spend their own money. With medicare, people spend someone else's money.
- Although producers in a normal market continuously search for ways to reduce costs, physicians and hospitals are under no such pressure. The success of a physician depends less on service to patients than on meeting requirements of third-party reimbursement formulas. Hospitals are granted global budgets that aren't a function of the services they provide.
- Innovation and technological change in a normal market are viewed as good for consumers, but government is hostile to new technologies because of their high prices.

With medicare, people acting in their own self-interest isn't desirable. Patients overconsume, driving up costs. Doctors overprovide, further increasing costs. Institutions resist change. The attempts to compensate for these tendencies — bureaucratic rule making — generate new perverse incentives.

Health care reform, then, should focus on undoing this mess. Rather than trying to find new ways to regulate people's behaviour, the goal should be to create a system with the proper incentives.

6.3 Back to Basics: Health Insurance

What is "medicare"? The question is a touch tricky. Medicare is a common yet inaccurate term, for it doesn't refer to an easily identifiable government program. Of course, we all have a pretty good idea of what the term means. A description of it might note that medicare covers many health services, that it is provincially administered, and that the federal government contributes to its financing. A health analyst would probably define the term using language such as "medicare is a state-financed health insurance plan" (Deber 1726). This is a straightforward definition that is often repeated.

But is medicare health "insurance"? It may seem so at first. Medicare, after all, means that the cost of health services isn't directly borne by the patient. People sometimes say that health services are "free." Such a claim is untrue. A visit to the doctor isn't free. The doctor gets paid by a third party (the government). Medicare thus seems like insurance: a certain amount of money is paid to the state, which covers expenses incurred.

But the idea of insurance has been distorted in health care. Insurance is meant to protect people in times of unforeseen or catastrophic events: automobile insurance (for car accidents), life insurance (for death), fire and casualty insurance (for damage to property), and disability insurance (for physical injury). There are more exotic examples — Lloyd's of London insures everything from the launch of satellites into space to warships entering the Persian Gulf.

One of the most common types of insurance is for houses. Although policies differ, most homeowners have a basic plan that protects them against the cost of repair after some type of disaster: a fire or a tree falling on the house, and so on. Financially, the purchase of insurance makes sense: the predictable cost of insurance is relatively small compared to the large and unpredictable cost of repair.

But medicare does more than just protect us against the cost of health care after a serious car accident or a lengthy bout with cancer. Medicare covers the costs associated with checkups, X-rays, and even frivolous visits to an emergency room. Medicare covers nearly all health care expenses.

Such coverage comes at a steep price. Imagine if a homeowner has insurance that covers all home expenses. Fire damage would be covered, but so would house painting, window washing, recarpeting, wallpapering, and cleaning. Under such circumstances, how often would the homeowner get the house cleaned? Often. How frequently would he or she redecorate? Frequently. Thus, the cost of the insurance would be vastly more expensive than a simple plan for catastrophes. The same applies to auto insurance. How much more would premiums be if insurance covered gasoline, oil changes, and paint jobs for nicks and scratches?

The same is true of our health "insurance" — because it covers nearly all health care expenses, taxpayers must shell out billions of dollars each year. The average working Canadian pays roughly 21¢ of every dollar earned for this all-inclusive insurance (see Clemens and Ramsay

5–7). This means that Canadians earning $35,000 a year pay $7,350 for medicare. Of course, part of this amount goes toward caring for the elderly and the chronically ill, but a large share goes toward paying for an inefficient system. Here again there's a perverse incentive to over-consume: because we know we're paying handsomely for medicare, we like to get our dollar's worth.

The problem occurs because medicare covers both catastrophic health expenses and discretionary spending. As discussed in chapter 4, the "free" nature of health care in Canada means that the doctor-patient relationship is corrupted and that institutional providers are uncompetitive. The only way to address these problems is to allow people to have more control over their health expenses. In short, discretionary spending must be divorced from catastrophic expenses: people should be covered in extreme situations but left to pay for minor problems.

Such a move would be a dramatic departure from health care re-forms to date, which have focused on restricting the supply of health care. Every province, from Ralph Klein's conservative Alberta to Roy Romanow's socialist Saskatchewan, has embarked on a similar pre-scription:

- restricting access to specialists,
- reducing the number of medical graduates,
- closing hospital beds,
- deinsuring certain services,
- restricting physician billing, and
- limiting the use of high-tech equipment.

The list doesn't end here. By trying to reduce supply, provincial govern-ments have taken an increasingly active role in our health care system — intervention needed, we are told, to help control costs.

But there's an alternative: allow individuals to make their own health care decisions. The reform would thus focus not on supply but on demand. The proposal is as simple as it is far-reaching. Canadians have long taken health care for granted. They have accepted that health care ought to be "free" and readily available. Hence, they have assumed that such a system means no tough decisions need to be made. If the doctor suggests that you need an X-ray, you have no reason not to get an X-ray.

But it's not as though decisions aren't made. They are simply made by other people. You don't need to think about the cost of an X-ray, but the Ministry of Health does. You don't worry about the cost of visiting walk-in clinics or lengthy hospital stays, but these costs add up.

Economists speak of the rationing of health care. Given that people's demands far outstrip supply even in the wealthiest nations, services must somehow be rationed. In Canada, rationing is achieved through restricting supply. Do people stay too long in hospitals? Then reduce the number of hospital beds. Do people get too many MRI scans? Then don't buy MRI machines. In many ways, rationing is achieved through waiting lists.

This approach may seem satisfactory, but it isn't. Consider that government reforms aren't designed for the individual case. It may make sense, say, to restrict the number of frivolous cases at an emergency room. Good luck trying to work that idea into policy. No, government reforms focus on the system. If emergency room use is expensive and many of the cases are deemed frivolous, then the number of emergency rooms is reduced. This is an arbitrary and unsatisfactory method of rationing care. Decisions are not made with intelligence and foresight. In the long run, the outcomes are far less clear. Cost control may be achieved, but many unintended consequences may develop — the exodus of physicians, for instance.

Demand-side reform would be very different. People would be empowered to make their own decisions about diagnostic tests, treatments, and hospital stays — and face, to some degree, the financial consequences. If you want the X-ray, fine, but you are going to have to pay for it.

"Consumer empowerment," as some proponents term it, may seem too radical. True, it would deal with the shortcomings of medicare, but at what cost? What about the poor and the chronically diseased? In our attempt to improve a mediocre health care system available to all, should we embrace a proposal that would result in quality health care for only a select few? No.

As with food, clothing, and shelter, it is possible to allow individual decision making and to address the needs of the less fortunate. More importantly, overhauling the financing of the system is likely the only way to save medicare. Consider the alternatives.

ALTERNATIVE I
More Money

Purpose: to reduce waiting lists.

Most Canadians accept that medicare has its share of problems, but far-reaching reforms are difficult to implement. No surprise, then, that the no-brainer option has become so popular: the system is under-funded and just needs more money.

Unions are particularly vocal on this point. But spending more on this social program isn't just a popular rallying cry in the union halls; it receives approval on Main Street. Allocating more money for health care has become the dominant idea about how to save medicare. As noted in chapter 2, the Liberals and the Reformers both agree that more money must be spent on the system.

The belief that the "new" funding will make a difference stems from the widely held perception that health care has been gutted in the 1990s. That perception is false — spending has never been higher in Canadian history than it is today. As noted in the introduction, total spending rose roughly 33% from 1990 to 1998 (before the federal "health care" budget of 1999).

Figures are easily manipulated — spending comparisons can be expressed on a per person basis or as total expenditure. But in this case, the presentation doesn't much matter. According to the data of the Canadian Institute for Health Information, total and per capita spending are both at all-time highs. As much as government politicians crow about reinvesting in health care and opposition politicians demand that more be done to put money back into it, we close the decade with a historic high.

And no wonder. For all the talk of deep cuts, health care spending increased every year this decade. On a per capita basis, spending dropped only one year this decade — in 1995. Spending that year, incidentally, didn't plummet by 10 or 20%. It fell by 0.1%. But what about inflation? Increases beat inflation each year except in 1995 and 1996.

Consider Ontario. It's commonly believed that the government under Premier Bob Rae spent generously on health care. With Premier Mike Harris at the helm, people assume a tight-fisted policy. But public spending per person has grown more in the first three years of Harris's government than in Rae's last three years in office.

But even if spending is up, wouldn't more money help? The argument has its charm. Proponents have a seductive logic: "Is there a long waiting time for CT scans? Then buy more CT scanners!"

But more money doesn't necessarily result in better health care. One crude measure of health care delivery is waiting times, and according to the Fraser Institute study they have never been longer in Canada despite the high spending.

Provincial comparisons also yield interesting results (see Ramsay and Walker, *Waiting* 17). Saskatchewan has the longest waits in the country — four months from family doctor to treatment. Yet that province's spending per person ranks third in Canada. British Columbia, the biggest spender per person, had a wait time of 12.6 weeks. Alberta ranked midpack on total spending and ninth on public spending (a full 20% below British Columbia's expenditure), but it had a wait time of 12.4 weeks.

Even if governments commit themselves to funding medicare by buckets full of money, the reality is that large cash infusions only buy the system a limited amount of time for survival. Demographic and technological trends suggest that a billion dollars or two just won't matter half a decade down the line.

Even now, when medicare consumes 21¢ of every dollar earned by working Canadians, the system is failing. As the population ages, demands on the system will dramatically grow. As noted in chapter 5, projections of future taxation rates needed to support medicare suggest unworkably high rates (94.5% in 2040, according to the Office of the Superintendent of Financial Services).

"More money for medicare" may make a good political slogan, but it's not a meaningful solution. The system must be made more efficient, but unfortunately this won't happen within the present framework.

ALTERNATIVE 2

Modest User Fees

Purpose: to limit patient overconsumption.

Currently, user fees are prohibited by the Canada Health Act. A province that chooses to implement even modest fees for services thus risks financial punishment. User fees, however, have been widely touted as a solution to our health care woes. Prominent politicians — former prime minister Kim Campbell, Alberta premier Ralph Klein, and former Quebec premier Daniel Johnson, to name a few — have favoured the idea. The Quebec National Assembly even passed a bill into law that allowed a user fee of five dollars for inappropriate use of emergency rooms in the province. (Because of the Canada Health Act restriction, the law exists on the books but has never been enforced.)

By and large, user fees have been argued in vague principle but not in any implementable form.[3] Such an approach may be politically shrewd — most ideas are more popular in principle than in detailed form. But because the concept of user fees remains murky, it's not clear what the term really means. Would such fees apply to all health care services (even emergencies) or only to certain ones? If only certain services, which ones? Would everyone pay these fees or only higher-income citizens? Would the fees represent a flat rate for a service or a portion of the overall cost?

These questions may seem picky. Some supporters of the idea urge us to agree on the basic concept and to work out the details later. The problem is that the potential benefits and drawbacks of implementing user fees depend very much on these details. A fee of five dollars for inappropriate use of an emergency room, for example, isn't likely to produce dramatic cost savings.

For the sake of analysis, let's consider percentage-based user fees of 25% for basic services. Such a proposal builds on the "supervalue phenomenon," exemplified by a western Canadian grocery chain that decided to break into the Winnipeg market. The chain built a large store with a diverse range of products: exotic foods, electronics, magazines from around the world, and enough fatty foods to make any dietitian cringe. To keep overall costs down, the company decided not to offer a bagging service. Instead, customers were given plastic shopping bags in which to pack their own groceries. The bags were free, and customers could use as many as they wished. The idea behind this approach was that labour costs could be kept down and grocery prices could remain competitive.

Unfortunately, people took to the yellow bags. After all, they were free — and useful. So the purchaser of a loaf of bread took five bags. Yellow bags became packed with other yellow bags.

The store decided to implement a modest user fee of four cents a bag. Even though the fee was small, the result was startling. People began to bring their old bags back. Others opted to use canvas bags. And most paused a moment to consider how many bags they really needed at the checkout. In short, even very modest user fees provide an incentive to economize. This we can term the supervalue phenomenon.

People intuitively understand this phenomenon. Every time they reach for their wallets, they hesitate. It's why they clip coupons for Sunkist oranges, buy shampoo at Walmart, or look for flats of yogurt at Costco. And, as noted in chapter 4, this phenomenon applies to health care.

Between 1968 and 1971, Saskatchewan charged modest user fees for medical services. A visit to the physician, for example, was $1.50. These charges resulted in a six percent drop in the use of physician services (the supervalue phenomenon). The Saskatchewan experience compares well with the findings of the RAND Health Insurance Experiment, in which the percentage of the user fee had a great effect on overall expenditures. The group charged no user fee consumed far more services than the group with the 25% charge. In other words, modest user fees do temper overconsumption. Implementing user fees, then, would be a step in the right direction. Dr. Martin Zelder, an economist whose PhD thesis was supervised by Nobel Laureate Gary Becker, suggests that total health care spending could be reduced by as much as $15 billion a year were 25% user fees charged.

Such fees, however, do little to better the overall system. They may reduce, for example, the number of misuses of an emergency room in a hospital, but they hardly provide an incentive for the hospital to operate more efficiently. In other words, user fees do nothing to promote competition and efficiency in the health care system.

ALTERNATIVE 3
Two-Tiered Medicare

Purpose: to free up resources within the system.

Like the concept of user fees, that of a two-tiered health care system conflicts with the Canada Health Act. Nevertheless, some analysts believe that allowing people to opt out of the public system and buy private insurance for private health care delivery is a solution to the woes of medicare. Dr. Grant Hill, the Official Opposition's health critic, has pushed the idea on occasion.

Allowing private sector health care delivery could take on a variety of forms: people could "buy" certain services at their discretion —

such as hip-replacement surgery — but could still rely on the public system at other times (as in the United Kingdom), or people could opt out of the public system entirely and thus be barred from public care (Germany's definition of two-tiered health care).

Two-tiered health care has its attractions. For one thing, the long waiting lists associated with medicare would be reduced as patients opt for the faster, private treatment, thereby relieving pressure on the public system. It's difficult to estimate the extent to which people would opt out of medicare if they were allowed to do so, but private care in other countries serves as a useful reference — and the data suggest that the reduction in waiting lists would be significant. In Britain, for example, the private sector provides 20% of all elective surgeries, including 30% of all hip-replacement procedures and 20% of coronary bypass operations, according to Tim Evans of the Independent Healthcare Association (Gray, "NHS" 1488). In Germany, about 10% of the population is covered by private insurance (Ulrich 66).

A private system, then, would lessen the burden on the public system and thus be of use to both those who opt for it and the vast majority left in the public system — the fewer the people on a waiting list for treatment, after all, the shorter the wait. The British model is particularly attractive in that private sector delivery serves as a safety valve of sorts. When demand for a certain procedure rises to high levels marked by long waiting lists, the private system allows steam to be let off.

Perhaps the greatest attraction of a private system is the indirect effects on the public system. The collection of information in the private system relating to treatment utilizations, costs, and outcomes would help medicare's planners. And the transparency of the parallel private system would serve as a modest form of competition — not competition for funding (the private system would presumably be private) but competition in the sense that the private sector would be a point of comparison for medicare. Administrators, for instance, would have greater incentive to streamline if they knew that politicians were watching their results and comparing them with those of the private system. In a small way, this would be the Federal Express method of health care reform — by direct comparison, the courier forces the post office to be more accountable. Likewise, private clinics capable of offering day surgeries at low cost would make government officials wonder how such procedures could be offered in the most cost-effective manner in the public system.

A commonly voiced argument in favour of the concept — one that is perhaps closest to the hearts of proponents of the private option — has nothing to do with practical implications. Proponents wonder why the state infringes on the liberties of citizens when it comes to health care. In our society, it is commonly accepted that citizens have the right to spend their money basically as they please. If you dream of driving a Mercedes-Benz and you make the money to buy one, then best of luck — enjoy the power of German engineering. Health care may seem different in that it addresses a physical need rather than a material desire. But, again, no government official stops you from ordering a steak dinner at Hy's Steak Loft, even though cooking a chicken at home would be far cheaper and just as filling. Similarly, no such official prevents you from saving to buy a bigger house, even though the one you live in has ample space.

Yet, when it comes to health care, the Canada Health Act basically forbids people from spending as they please. It's ironic that private health care is allowed in countries supposedly less free than our own. A member of a British Columbia District Health Council, for example, argued vigorously against private sector health care but then left his position to do consulting work in China on establishing private hospitals (Day, telephone interview). Such stories aren't rare. Canada is the only major economy in the world in which it's illegal to sell private insurance for services covered by the public system.

The hypocrisy is clear. Notes Michael Walker of the Fraser Institute:

> If someone claims hot wax in your ears might cure a headache, they can advertise that and take your money for the procedure. But if you're on the waiting list for an MRI head scan, which could be six to eight weeks or longer, you're not allowed to use your own money to buy that service privately. (telephone interview)

The opponents of two-tiered health care respond angrily and passionately. They charge that private sector care would destroy the medicare system. But would allowing people to spend their own money more freely really result in a slippery slope where the rich get quality care and the poor fend for themselves? Such a charge is based on the assumption that, with a private system, many will opt out of the public system and then promptly refuse to pay for it. By this logic, the public system would wither on the vine. But the experiences of countries such as Germany and Britain indicate that the vast majority of people

— meaning the vast majority of voters — would still rely on the public system.

A parallel, private system isn't the archenemy of medicare that it has been portrayed as; indeed, it would serve a useful role. But a private system won't be the great saviour of medicare. The public system would largely remain an inefficient mess. True, some improvements to it would inevitably result, but the perverse incentives would continue to exist and ensure that billions of dollars are wasted.

ALTERNATIVE 4

Internal Markets

Purpose: to increase competitiveness between institutional providers of health care.

Within the confines of the Canada Health Act, perhaps medicare could be administered in a more efficient manner. While provincial governments have opted to increase government control over the health care system, some observers have argued that an alternative exists: greater competition. At first, this alternative may seem counterintuitive. Patients, after all, don't pay for the services they receive. Such an arrangement limits the potential for direct market competition. But many countries, including New Zealand and the United Kingdom, have attempted to create an internal market within the framework of a state-run and state-financed system (see Forget and Jérôme-Forget).

The concept of the internal market is based on distinguishing between purchasing health care services and providing these services. Purchasing and providing are two very different functions. The purchaser of a service is concerned with its cost, the need it satisfies, and its quality. The provider is financially dependent on satisfying the demands of the purchaser. (With global budgeting, there's no real purchaser, and providers are therefore relatively free to do as they please, with little concern for the communities they serve.) Internal market reforms seek to make the state the purchaser and the various publicly funded institutions the autonomous providers.[4]

Establishment of the Purchasers

Regional Health Authorities (RHAs) are created for specific geographic jurisdictions and funded on the basis of population. They are charged with determining the health care needs of the communities they serve and then purchasing the required services.

Establishment of the Providers

Hospitals and other institutions are freed from the constraints of government — both the numerous regulations and the public service contractual obligations. However, direct funding is terminated. Hospitals, or trusts as they are called, must compete for contracts from the RHAs.

In theory, an internal market system would replace the present hospital cartel with a dynamic group of hospitals, specialized clinics, day surgery centres, long-term-care facilities, home care services, and diagnostic testing centres competing for contracts.

In Britain and New Zealand, the internal market concept includes another level. Groups of family physicians are allowed to become fundholders. They agree to take care of a certain number of registered patients. In exchange, the DHAs directly grant them funds to pay for the basic medical needs of their patients, such as diagnostic testing, radiology, physiotherapy, day surgeries, and community nursing. The fundholders are then encouraged to buy the needed services from competing providers. If the fundholders are able to purchase the necessary services for less than the amount of money granted, the savings are rolled back into their clinics.[5] There's a strong incentive for physicians to shop around and get competitive offers.

Since the concept was originally debated in various academic circles in the 1980s, various countries have experimented with internal markets. And, although these countries have unique health care systems, they do have public health care systems that are compatible with Canada's medicare. The most ambitious internal market reforms (upon which the above ideas are based) have been undertaken in the National Health Service (United Kingdom).

Sir Richard Storey, chairman of York Health Services Trust, describes in an essay the dramatic changes that have occurred in his public hospital after the introduction of the reforms. He notes that cost-effective day surgeries have doubled — a change that "could never have been achieved under the old order: innovations of established best practice could take a leisurely decade or two" (85). Financial accountability has improved; support services (laundry and waste disposal) have been contracted out; and customer care is a higher priority (the hospital "has taken more soundings from the public in the last 12 months than in the last 12 years!" [84]). Storey believes that with the reforms people "get a better service" primarily because "many hospitals are genuinely competing with their neighbours. . . . [The] practical reality is that patients and those representing them are voting with their feet and money bags whither better treatments can be found" (87).

Stephen Pollard, a British Labour Party advisor and head of research at the Social Market Foundation, writes of these reforms that

> The overwhelming evidence . . . has been that the split works. It is more efficient, makes possible spending of greater resources on health care itself, and makes the provider more accountable to the purchaser, who now has real purchasing power. Many of the people pointing this out have been solid Labour supporters or advisors such as Julian Le Grand of the London School of Economics. (12)

In some senses, the NHS reforms have been successful. At least superficially, hospitals and other institutional providers are forced to improve their financial accountability. But the effects of the reforms have been limited. Studies suggest that many RHAs merely buy their services from hospitals as they have in the past — because of habit and fear of political embarrassment, many DHAs have effectively put their hospitals on global budgets (OECD, *Internal Markets* 18). Moreover, while waiting lists initially dropped after the reforms (in 1991, for instance, 200,000 people were on lists for procedures such as coronary bypass operations and hip replacements for at least two years; in 1996, no one waited that long [Gray, "NHS" 1487]), waits have since grown.

6.4 Up from Medicare

Each of the above alternatives seems like a step in the right direction but is ultimately unsatisfactory in itself. User fees temper demand but fail to address competitiveness. Internal markets introduce competitiveness but fall short in reducing excess demand. Two-tiered health care and increased funding improve the availability of health services but do little to address inefficiencies in the system. Each alternative would improve the system in the short term. British-style internal markets make more sense, for instance, than the central management that the provincial governments have uniformly embraced. Increased funding would reduce waiting lists, as would allowing private health insurance.

Some analysts advocate a mixture of these reforms: internal markets *and* user fees, two-tiered health care *and* more money, et cetera. Such a mixture would also be a marked improvement over the present batch of so-called reforms. The most worthwhile changes would probably be the legalization of private insurance and user fees. But the problems faced by medicare are profound, and they demand more than simple, short-term improvements. If the goal is to build a lasting, sustainable health care system based on the belief that patients deserve quality, accessible, cost-effective, timely, and patient-oriented care, then the entire system must be overhauled.

No matter how much Canadians want the present system to work, it will inevitably fail. The problem with medicare isn't that governments haven't experimented enough with micromanagement. The problem isn't that providers are compensated in an ineffective manner. And the problem isn't that more funds are needed. *The real problem with medicare is its utopian design.*

Reform of the system won't work unless its design is changed. Put another way, the doctor-patient relationship must be reestablished. The alternatives considered in this chapter do nothing to achieve this end — they only attempt to further manipulate supply and demand. The solutions to our health care problems won't be found in further tinkering. The easiest way to reestablish the doctor-patient relationship is through financial ties. Doctors must again be paid by their patients.

In many ways, the pathology of our health care system isn't unlike that of the old Soviet industry.[6] Many people remember the folly of the Soviet factory that turned out two left boots. Few, however, seem to remember the moral of the story. Because customers paid in soft currency, they took what they could get. They had no power to demand better. Because the factory was compensated in soft currency, they didn't need to worry about the customers' needs.

Reform, then, must be built on the principle that patients should pay directly for their health care.

There are still many questions to be answered. How can accessibility be maintained? Would catastrophic events lead to bankruptcy? Would the poorest citizens suffer? These concerns are effectively addressed with a system of medical savings accounts (outlined in the next chapter).

But the most important step toward renewing health care in this country is to accept that medicare is fundamentally flawed. As long as politicians cling to the notion that medicare has worked well in the past and that, with the right amount of tinkering, it will work well in the future, waiting lists will just get longer. These "reforms" have as much hope of succeeding as the alchemists had of making gold from lead.

Fortunately, there's a better way.

7

Why Choice and Freedom Work

"FORGET about practising medicine," a provincial health minister's assistant advised, "the real money's in health care consulting." No doubt — a consultant can fetch up to $1,500 a day.

Provincial governments are desperate for advice on how to reform our health care system. For over a decade, they have experimented with everything from bed closures to regional health boards, all in the name of "cost control." The results haven't been stellar. Waiting lists are long and growing. Hospital standards are lackadaisical. High-tech diagnostic machines are scarce. Talented physicians are leaving for the United States. The public is increasingly concerned.

What's a health minister to do? The answer may be found in a company from Indiana.

7.1 Looking to the Golden Rule

Based in Indianapolis, Golden Rule is an insurance company with some 1,300 employees. Like most American corporations, it provides its employees with health care coverage. In the early 1990s, management at Golden Rule had a problem: with expensive new technologies such as MRI scanners and powerful pharmaceuticals, the cost of health care was rising dramatically. The company had to find a way to save money on health care coverage.

Many companies in the United States have responded to this problem by looking to Health Maintenance Organizations (HMOs), which attempt to balance patients' needs with cost control. But many patients have found that cost control is more important to these companies than quality care. HMOs — like provincial governments in Canada — have sought to control costs by denying patients access to medical specialists, diagnostic tests, and hospital care.

Golden Rule decided that managed care may not be the best option. Why have a bureaucrat make decisions for its employees? The employees should make their own decisions. So in 1993 the company decided to experiment with a new type of health care coverage.

To ensure that a major illness wouldn't bankrupt an employee, Golden Rule provided catastrophic insurance — a policy that covered all expenses above $2,000 US a year. Thus, an employee hit by a bus or stricken with cancer wouldn't have to sell his house to pay for the medical bills. For minor health expenses such as yearly physicals, X-rays, and prenatal care, the company deposited $1,000 US in a special medical savings account, or MSA. When an employee needed minor medical attention, she simply paid for it from her MSA. For families, coverage began at $3,000 US, with $2,000 US put into the MSA.

Because the plan was new, Golden Rule decided to make it optional. Employees could either stick with their traditional insurance plan or choose the new plan. In 1993, most employees — some 80% in all — chose the MSA plan. Over the next half-decade, the popularity of the program grew. Today the MSA plan is the choice of 98% of employees.

The popularity of the program isn't surprising. When an employee wants to see a doctor, she doesn't have to fill out forms or get permission from an HMO bureaucrat. She simply goes to the doctor and pays for the visit using her MSA. As an incentive for the employee to spend wisely, Golden Rule allows money remaining in the account at the end of the year to be withdrawn and spent freely. For the average employee, this translated into a $1,000 US bonus per year.

MSAs also offer employees new choices. Since they have cash on hand to pay for health services, they can purchase preventive care. According to the vice-president's office, a full 20% of employees reported in 1994 that they purchased services they wouldn't have under the traditional insurance. Today the statistic is closer to 26%.

And, for the management of Golden Rule, medical savings accounts have meant a drop in health care costs. Major health expenses dropped in 1994 by 40% (Ferrara, "More" 9). This drop isn't surprising, for patients have an incentive to think before they use health services.

Consider the story of Shelli Johnson on the company's Web site. When a doctor told her that she needed several tests, she called the local hospital and was told the bill would be $785. Concerned by the high cost, she decided to shop around. Another hospital, it turned out, was willing to perform the necessary tests for only $114 — a saving of nearly $700. "If I hadn't had the medical savings account," Johnson wrote to her boss, "I would never have even thought to ask about the cost of the tests, not to mention thinking of shopping around for a better price."

★   ★   ★

There isn't a perfect solution to Canada's health care problem. Any proposal will have its share of drawbacks and complications. But Golden Rule's intelligent alternative isn't a bad place to start.

At first glance, Golden Rule may seem like an unusual place to turn to for health care ideas. Forget that many Canadians can't point out Indianapolis — or even Indiana — on a map. Forget that with a payroll of 1,300 Golden Rule isn't a particularly large company — and certainly tiny compared to Canada, with millions of people. Forget that employee-purchased health coverage seems very alien to people who associate health care with government financing. The fact is that the administration of Golden Rule faced a problem in the early 1990s that many other administrations have faced — other American companies and Canada's provinces. On the one hand, Golden Rule needed to contain costs. On the other hand, it wanted to provide quality health care for its employees. American corporations and Canadian governments have generally attempted to deal with this dilemma by taking decision making away from individuals and giving it to bureaucrats.

Amazingly, Golden Rule managed to come up with a way to provide its employees with both the health care coverage they wanted and the freedom to make their own decisions. The idea was so simple that it could have been written on the back of a postcard. For major illnesses, employees have catastrophic insurance. For minor expenses (what economists such as Ake Blomqvist refer to as "discretionary spending"), employees have money in an account to spend as they please, but they also have a strong incentive not to squander the money.

Is this the way to achieve a better health care system in Canada? Can we address the fundamental woes of medicare without having to settle hundreds of details such as the ideal number of hospitals or the best way to purchase laundry services? Maybe. The MSA concept is best understood by considering a couple of simple examples.

What if Widow Jones decides to have her bad cough checked out by a doctor? Under an MSA system, she would see her family physician, who would bill not the provincial government but Widow Jones directly. She wouldn't need to break her piggy bank; instead, she would draw money from her account, possibly using a debit card. She wouldn't have to fill out forms or seek permission from a government bureaucrat.

What if Mr. Smith is hit by a bus? When humans and buses collide, the former tend to fare poorly. Mr. Smith would require a lengthy hospital stay, surgery, countless tests, and physiotherapy. Of course, all of this would come with a high price tag. But under an MSA system, he would be covered by catastrophic health insurance. When a house burns down, the insured owner isn't required to pay for every new door handle and window pane in the replacement home. Likewise, Mr. Smith wouldn't be left with a hefty bill for all the medical services he has received.

Clearly, these simple examples provide only a basic understanding. In this chapter, we will look at some of the more interesting aspects of the MSA concept: the restoration of the doctor-patient relationship, the creation of a sustainable health care system, and its implications for preventive medicine.

But already it should be clear that medical savings accounts are worth considering. For one thing, the MSA concept passes the most basic criterion for a decent health care system: "the house test." This is the requirement that no person who falls ill should lose his or her house paying for the medical bills. Golden Rule employees may lose their houses because of bad hands (and a great deal of whisky) during poker games or investments in Bre-X but not because of steep medical bills; for those, they have catastrophic insurance.

7.2 MSAs: Nine Questions and Answers

1. How Does an MSA Work?

Health care financed through medical savings accounts is built on two cornerstones: the MSA (which we will refer to as the "account"), and an insurance for catastrophic illness. The account is just like a bank account — it contains a certain amount of money that can be drawn to cover minor health expenses. The insurance covers catastrophic expenses — thus, it doesn't kick in until a high threshold (deductible) had been reached.

When we speak of MSAs, we really mean three different levels of payment. First, health services are paid for by the money in the account. For instance, a man sees his family physician for an annual checkup at a cost, say, of $15. This amount would be paid from the account. Second, if the money in the account is exhausted, the individual must pay out of pocket to a point. Hence, a woman who sees many doctors for minor illnesses may eventually have to take her cheque-book to the doctor's office. Third, when patients are really sick (e.g., a man is struck by a bus and forced to spend six months in a hospital), the high-deductible insurance kicks in. It prevents a catastrophic illness from becoming a catastrophic personal expense.

As a financial incentive to spend wisely, account holders are given options for using the money remaining in the account at the end of the year. Depending on the MSA model, account holders can either roll their balances into next year's account, thereby gaining greater future buying power, or withdraw the money to spend as they please.

The Fraser Institute advocates a form of MSAs, which it refers to as Medical Premium Accounts, in *Healthy Incentives: Canadian Health Reform in an International Context*. The approach isn't intended to save the health care system money — it aims, instead, for governments to spend health care dollars differently. Take, for example, a single man aged 25 (Ramsay, McArthur, and Walker 190). In British Columbia, the government spends on his health care an average of $649 a year. Under the proposed system, the government would still spend the $649. The authors of *Healthy Incentives* argue that $298 of that money should go toward a mandatory insurance with a $1,000 deductible. The young man would have the rest of the money ($351) to put into an account and spend at his discretion. If he spends all the money in the account — that is, his medical bills exceed $351 — he is responsible for paying expenses out of pocket until he reaches the $1,000 deductible, at which time the insurance would cover the cost of services.

The Consumer Policy Institute offers its own plan, termed Health Allowances. A 30-year-old man, for instance, would be given an allowance of $416. His mandatory insurance would kick in at $520 — so, if his health care expenses run over $416, he's out of pocket for up to $104. The numbers were worked out by Milliman and Robertson, one of the leading health actuarial firms in the United States, which conducted a comprehensive feasibility study for the Consumer Policy Institute. The institute also envisions that certain preventive health measures would remain free, thus encouraging Canadians to prevent illnesses (Solomon).

Both models offer Canadians relative freedom in spending the money in their accounts. Money could be spent on physiotherapy, alternative medicines, and other health services not currently covered by medicare. And both models adjust for age, gender, and health. An elderly woman with diabetes, after all, requires more health services than a young, healthy man. Thus, she would be granted more money for her account.

There is another MSA model, though it has been neither researched nor promoted by any Canadian institution. Rather than have the government grant each individual or family a certain amount of money, people would be allowed to put a tax-free portion of their income in MSAs. Because the government would no longer have to fund the bulk of health expenses, taxes could be cut substantially.

Although the three models differ in details, the basic principle is the same. Provincial governments wouldn't spend money for you on health care. You would spend money on health care for yourself.

It's interesting to note the differences in reasoning offered by the various MSA advocates. For the Fraser Institute, MSAs offer a way to better organize health care in Canada. The institute sees consumer empowerment as increasing both personal responsibility and competition. For the Consumer Policy Institute, MSAs are about making Canadians healthier. Consumer empowerment, it argues, increases people's wellness because it gives them greater control over their lives.

MSAs attract a great diversity of supporters in both Canada and other countries. Proponents of alternative medicine, free-market economists, libertarian individualists, profit-minded corporations, employee-minded unions, believers in preventive health, demographics-obsessed public policy gurus, consumers seeking choice — all these groups see some value in MSAs. No wonder. MSAs offer people something a government-managed health care system can't: choice.

Let's review the three core principles of MSAs.

1. People pay directly for minor health expenses — first out of their accounts, then out of their pockets.
2. For catastrophic expenses, people are covered by a high-deductible insurance.
3. There's a financial incentive for people to spend wisely.

2. *Would People Neglect Their Health?*

MSAs require that people make health-related decisions for themselves. And who better than you to make decisions about your health care? It's easy to see the advantage of such an arrangement. There's not only increased autonomy but also an increased incentive to *not* rush to the doctor for every illness, because you get to keep any unspent money in your account.

But the MSA concept has its share of critics. Providing people with an incentive not to rush to the doctor for every minor ailment may prove to be a double-edged sword. Yes, abuse of medicare would be reduced. But at what cost? The lonely senior citizen may no longer use her family physician's office for afternoon socializing because of the financial disincentive, but will others begin to neglect their health? Will the neighbour two doors down — who buys his salsa by the gallon to save money — avoid getting a minor problem checked out until it's a major problem? Health care, these critics suggest, is so complex that people can't be expected to know their own needs. Does the average person really know the difference between a flu and meningitis, a mole and melanoma, heart burn and heart attack? Encouraged not to use the system, won't patients underuse health care? Won't such underuse result in higher long-term costs?

Raisa Deber, a professor in the Department of Health Administration at the University of Toronto, argues exactly this point: small problems will be neglected if people have a financial incentive not to see a doctor: "The whole idea behind health promotion — making people healthy instead of treating them when they're sick — is that you don't want people to come in until they have a heart attack or a diabetic coma" (qtd. in Coutts, "Group").

The argument is persuasive, but it isn't supported by the data. As discussed earlier, the California think tank RAND tracked 2,000 families over eight years in a study that cost more than $100 million US (1984). The study compared the health and the health care spending of two groups: one with free health care, the other with user fees for services. The result? People on the free plan were significantly more expensive but in the end no more healthy than those on the user fee plan. The lack of difference in overall health status indicates that patients are able to make intelligent health care choices when provided with a financial incentive to do so.

There's a further argument in favour of MSAs: they may actually make people healthier than the present system. Because account holders would have cash on hand, they could utilize more preventive health care than they currently do. The experience of Golden Rule employees supports this argument: a quarter of the people with MSAs reported that they used preventive care they previously hadn't used.

"Prevention" is a vague term that has been manipulated by different groups to mean different things. The evidence, however, is that health promotion programs do prevent health problems. A two-year random trial involving 43,000 employees of Dupont found that sick days could be reduced by 14% through a health education initiative. Such a result isn't isolated. In a recent article in *Health Affairs*, former US surgeon general C. Everett Koop and four coauthors reviewed 32 programs and found that such efforts generally reduced health insurance claims by 20%.

The present health care system doesn't do much to encourage preventive care. By making money for such services readily available and by increasing people's consciousness of health care costs, MSAs could change this disincentive.

3. *What Are the Immediate Benefits of MSAs?*

Perhaps the single most important benefit of medical savings accounts would be their effect on the doctor-patient relationship.

As discussed in Chapter 4, under medicare at present the doctor-patient relationship is distorted. For the patient, there's no need to think about cost. As a result, patients tend to overuse health services — they see doctors too often, they request too many tests, and they stay in hospitals too long. For the doctor, the impetus to serve the needs of patients is replaced by the impetus to serve a fee schedule. Doctors thus have an incentive to overprovide health services. Provincial health care reforms — really a euphemism for limiting the availability of health services to patients — have attempted to offset these incentives.

MSA-based reforms would restore the doctor-patient relationship. Patients would be held financially accountable for their decisions. Every dollar spent on a test would be one dollar less in a patient's account. The doctor, in turn, would receive compensation from patients, not from a provincial government. The doctor-patient relationship would be reinvigorated with financial ties.

4. *Can the Doctor-Patient Relationship Be Restored under the Present Structure?*

Some analysts argue that a simpler method of restoring the doctor-patient relationship would be to change the way physicians are compensated. If the fee-for-service approach encourages doctors to overprovide services, then wouldn't it make sense to put doctors on salaries? A surprisingly large number of people would say yes, people ranging from health policy experts — *Strong Medicine* authors Michael Rachlis and Carol Kushner, for instance, are bullish on changing physician compensation — to popular authors such as David Foot and Daniel Stoffman of *Boom, Bust, and Echo* fame.

Proponents of this view offer two different approaches. First, doctors could just be put on flat salaries, presumably influenced by the number of hours worked and the level of training. Second, capitation could be introduced, whereby doctors would be paid according to the number of patients they take care of, with patients' ages and health influencing compensation.

The problem is that any salary-based change to physician compensation would almost surely affect the work ethic. A small study comparing the work of pediatric resident physicians on fee for service and those on salary found just this (Hickson, Altemeier, and Perrin). The fee-for-service physicians scheduled more visits, provided better continuity of care, and were responsible for fewer emergency room visits. The study may have been small, but the findings are consistent with the experiences of countries where physicians are salaried. In Sweden, for example, physicians are salaried — and it has the reputation of having the least productive doctors in Europe. Margit Gennser, a member of the Swedish parliament, reports that it isn't unusual for Swedish doctors to see only six to 10 patients a day (61).

Capitation has been the standard method of paying family physicians in the British health care system for 50 years. Yet the United Kingdom has many of the same problems with the National Health Service as Canada does with medicare — two examples are waiting lists and a dearth of high-tech equipment. Perhaps this isn't so surprising. Capitation — or, for that matter, flat salaries — have little effect on the way patients use the health care system. A salaried doctor may have less desire to overprovide services, but her patients will still be tempted to overconsume. Only medical savings accounts offer a real way to reestablish the doctor-patient relationship.

5. *What Are the Long-Term Implications of MSAs?*

Medical savings accounts offer a long-term advantage over the present system: sustainability.

Although the effects of an aging population are seldom discussed in Canada today, this demographic shift threatens to bankrupt our social safety net. As observed in Chapter 5, an aging population has profound implications for future health care usage. It's common sense, after all, that a 70 year old sees a doctor more often than a 20 year old, and studies confirm this assumption. From a societal point of view, these implications are far-reaching: as the percentage of elderly Canadians doubles to a quarter of the total population over the next four decades, more Canadians will demand health services, yet the number of working Canadians will decrease relatively. Canada's health care *Titanic* is heading full-speed toward a financial iceberg.

The problem is that the present system is financed — to use a technical term — on a "pay-as-you-go" basis. Today's medical bills are footed by today's taxpayers: governments fund health care out of general tax revenue. Tomorrow, when there are fewer taxpayers and more health care consumption, it will be more difficult for taxpayers to foot the medical bills. Writing in *Fraser Forum* on European health care, Paul Belien, the research director for the Centre for the New Europe, explains that

> All of the European systems, even the present private ones, are financed on a pay-as-you-go basis whereby today's healthy and young foot the bill for today's sick and elderly. The costs of the present generation are shifted to the next generation, but this has become unsustainable given our present demographic evolution. (12)

The same situation exists in Canada — the pay-as-you-go approach to health care will inevitably result in disaster. The alternative is to have people save for the health care needs of their elderly years. Belien explains the necessary switch: "we should transform our health care system from [a] pay-as-you-go system into systems financed by means of capitalization. In a capitalization system, the money that is put in the system today is set aside for future needs" (12). Because MSAs encourage people to save money, they provide capitalization — just what Canadians need to see baby boomers reach and live beyond retirement.

It's possible to hypothesize what would happen over the next 40 years if MSAs were in place (see epilogue). Given the incentive to spend wisely, today's middle-aged Canadians would spend the money in their accounts frugally, allowing money to accrue over the years. The savings would grow, creating a health care nest egg. In their elderly years, these new seniors would have to pay more for catastrophic insurance — the possibility of catastrophic illness is much higher, of course, for seniors — but they would have savings to cover the expense. And they could afford services such as home care in their twilight years.

The health care system itself would change. Given the financial incentives to serve patients' needs, health care would naturally move from its expensive focus on acute care and shift into catering to the needs of an elderly clientele — cost-effective home care.

The present course of medicare contrasts sharply with this scenario. With an aging population, resources will continue to be stretched. Eventually, governments will have to raise taxes to cover expenses. But the baby boom generation is too large — waiting lists will grow, and services will be increasingly inaccessible. If we find it unacceptable today that an elderly parent has to wait in pain for an entire year to get a hip replacement, how will we feel when we have to wait a couple of years or longer for the surgery?

6. What about the Poor?

Many supporters of medicare have argued that any change to the system would be detrimental to the poor. There is some evidence, in fact, that certain health care reforms may adversely affect the poor.

The RAND Health Insurance Experiment, for instance, concluded that user fees caused poor patients suffering from high blood pressure to neglect their condition. This wasn't the only such study. In 1982, California substantially changed its health coverage for the poor. When the effects of these changes were studied, researchers concluded that the poor suffered from a significant increase in uncontrolled hypertension (see the two studies by Lurie et al.).

Why was high blood pressure so problematic? First, given that the poor are preoccupied with basic needs such as putting food on the table, it's not surprising that dealing with long-term problems such as hypertension would have lower priority. Second, these studies were done at a time when the effects of hypertension weren't well understood among the general population. Both factors played a role. Not surprisingly, the RAND Health Insurance Experiment researchers recommended that "a one-time screening examination" for high blood pressure be made free and available (Newhouse and the Insurance Experiment Group 243).

The Consumer Policy Institute suggests that all preventive health measures — such as regular blood pressure checks — should remain free (Solomon). Cost-free prevention is likely unnecessary. After all, a well-designed MSA system makes it easy for the poorest citizens to get quality health care — they can be directly granted money by the state for their health care needs. And those with special medical needs — chronic conditions such as hypertension or diabetes — could be granted more money.

In fact, the poor may well be better off under an MSA system for three reasons. First, MSAs would allow them to pay for the many services that provincial governments have either deinsured or tagged with stiff user fees. A poor Albertan is required to pay for both a visit to an optometrist and crutches should a leg be on the mend. An MSA would provide him or her with the money to cover these expenses. Second, MSAs would give Canada's poor the cash necessary to purchase certain types of preventive medicine. And third, an MSA system would be sustainable over the long term. Those who will be hurt the most if our public system collapses are the poorest citizens, for they are the least able to pay for health care.

7. Would MSAs Pass the Five Pillars Test?

As described in Chapter 6, a health care system should be judged by its ability to meet five criteria, the five pillars. Although the present health care system doesn't pass the test, an MSA-based system would. Let's consider each criterion.

Patient orientation. Health services would have to make patients their priority or face the wrath of an empowered consumer. With MSAs, patients would pay for their own health care. Thus, decision making would rest not with bureaucrats but with patients. At the most basic level, then, physicians would serve patients, not the state billing schedule.

Accessibility. Catastrophic insurance would prevent major medical expenses from becoming financial catastrophes. And, since the state would directly help the poorest citizens by providing them with health care dollars for their accounts, no citizen would be deprived of the health care needed.

Quality. As with any system that promotes competition, the clinics, hospitals, and other providers of health care services would have a financial incentive to improve the services to attract patients. Health care providers would naturally want to invest in the latest technologies, innovate their delivery of health services, and ensure proper standards of quality.

Timeliness. In areas where patient demand outstrips the available supply — for example, high-tech diagnostic equipment — clinics and hospitals would have an incentive to invest in the needed equipment. After all, patients' needs translate into opportunities for health care providers in an MSA system.

Cost effectiveness. Because patients would be held financially responsible for their actions, they would have a strong incentive to become more informed and then shop around before making health care decisions. This effort would reduce the number of unnecessary tests and procedures. And it would force health care providers to streamline — excessive administration and inflated employee wages hurt competitiveness.

8. Are MSAs Used Anywhere?

Looking to the Far East, we can see a country that is testing the theories. Plagued by rising health care costs, this country's government recently embarked on an experiment in medical savings accounts. The results are of interest.

Here's how the program works. Individuals are required to put six percent of their wages into a medical savings account. A further five percent must be put into a common fund, the "social risk pool." When an individual uses a health service, he or she pays out of the MSA. Any amount left over at the end of the year is rolled into the following year's account.

When funds are exhausted, individuals must pay from their own pockets, up to five percent of their annual income. Anything above this level is considered catastrophic and is largely paid from the community's social risk pool. If a worker is hit by a bus and medical expenses run to two-and-a-half times his annual salary, he will actually be responsible for expenses amounting to a quarter of his annual salary.

Although the experiment is still new, impressive results are already being realized. In one year, total health spending fell by a staggering 24.6%. This result is all the more remarkable given that in neighbouring cities, where citizens still enjoy "free" health care, spending grew by 35–40%. Interestingly, savings weren't derived from fewer hospital stays or physician visits. The savings came from decreased use of diagnostic tests and expensive pharmaceuticals. The number of X-rays, for example, declined by more than half.

What innovative, forward-looking country is this? China. And the experiment involves five million citizens. This isn't an endorsement of the Chinese model per se — it relies heavily on government regulation of physicians' fees and public administration of hospitals. Nevertheless, the results suggest that even a restrictive form of medical savings accounts can yield dramatic results.

Other countries have adopted the use of medical savings accounts. The country with the most developed system of MSAs is Singapore (see Asher). In 1955, the government of Singapore introduced a compulsory savings program to allow citizens to better save for their retirement. Although the accounts belong to individuals, employees and employers are required by law to contribute to the Central Provident Fund (CPF).

Originally, the compulsory savings had nothing to do with health care. The system was primarily designed to ensure that citizens can retire with an adequate pension, though employees can withdraw money from the funds to purchase a home, buy life insurance, or pay for college education. The system works, in some ways, like a mandatory RRSP. Individuals also have some flexibility in how the money in their funds is invested, and deposits and withdrawals can be made tax free. Funds can be withdrawn at retirement, in the event of permanent disability, or should a citizen emigrate from the country.

The original impetus for the mandatory savings was to provide some capitalization for Singapore's pensions. Like many Western nations, Singapore has an aging population.[1] Recognizing that the shifting demographics would have a profound effect on both pensions and health care, the government expanded the program in 1984 to cover certain health services.

Today a portion of the mandatory contributions for each individual goes toward a Medisave account. Like so many aspects of life in Singapore, use of the Medisave accounts is subject to regulations and restrictions. A patient requiring a hospital stay can choose either a private or a public hospital and pay for the stay out of his or her Medisave account. On the other hand, most out-patient services don't qualify for withdrawals from these accounts. In recent years, some restrictions have been relaxed.

After a few years of experimentation, the Singapore government decided that more needed to be done to ensure that citizens had good access to health care. So, in 1990, the government introduced a catastrophic insurance option, the Medishield program. According to age, Singapore citizens can now purchase a high-deductible insurance with the funds in their Medisave accounts.

And the commitment to accessibility doesn't end with Medishield. To assist the poorest of citizens, the government established Medifund, an endowed fund to help those with limited resources. And many public hospital wards receive subsidies. Ward B2 patients in a Singapore public hospital, for example, pay only 36% of the cost of their hospitalization — but they must share a room with five other people. In contrast, Ward A patients are cared for in private rooms — but they must foot the entire bill from their Medisave accounts.

It's difficult to judge the success of Singapore's health care system. For one thing, information on Medifund patients is sorely lacking (see Asher). Still, some crude analysis can be done. The wages of doctors in Singapore are on par with those of doctors in the United States and higher than those of doctors in Canada (see Hsiao). Diagnostic medical equipment, such as CT and MRI scanners, is more abundant in Singapore than in Canada. And — while we shouldn't pin too much importance on international comparisons — Singapore has achieved an accessible health care system while spending only 3.1% of its GDP.

Both Singapore and China recognize that there is value in individual choice when it comes to health care. If these two countries, with their long authoritarian histories, can recognize this value, why can't Canada?

The public and private sectors in the United States have also become laboratories in the MSA experiment. Many employers — both large and small — are choosing to provide employees with medical savings accounts for insurance coverage rather than traditional insurance (see Ferrara, "More"). This choice isn't surprising. For employers, MSAs are a cost-effective way of providing health coverage. For employees, they offer health care coverage that isn't dictated by HMO bureaucrats.

Perhaps the best example of MSAs at work in the United States is at Golden Rule, as discussed above. Policy analyst Peter Ferrara provides other examples of MSAs in the United States (see "More"; all figures in US dollars).

- *Windham Hospital.* The Connecticut hospital with 1,000 employees switched from a plan with no deductible or user fee to a plan with a $500 deductible, and the employer put up $520 in a medical savings account for each employee. Prior to the switch, employees used health services 35% more often than other members of the community. Under the MSA plan, employees use the services to the same extent as the community average. The hospital has thus reduced projected health costs by about 50% (13).

- *United Mine Workers Union*. Because of the appeal of MSAs, the union negotiated MSA-style health coverage for the 15,000 employees of Bituminous Coal Operators Association. Miners are provided with a high-deductible insurance and a $1,000 bonus at the start of each year to be used for health expenses (15–16).

- *Quaker Oats*. The cereal manufacturer provides workers with a high-deductible insurance. The company also deposits $300 in a medical savings account. Over the first 10 years of the plan, health costs grew by 6.3% annually. In the rest of the country, growth rates were more than 10% (14).

- *Jersey City*. Employees of Jersey City, New Jersey, can choose between traditional insurance and an MSA plan. An insurance policy covers all expenses over $1,500 for individuals and $2,000 for families. The city then puts $1,500 and $2,000, respectively, in the accounts of these employees. Workers can withdraw all unspent MSA money at the end of the year. Even though workers can withdraw up to $2,000 a year, the city finds that, because of reduced administrative costs, medical expenses are lower with the MSA plan (15).

The differences are significant. Deductibles for the catastrophic insurance policies vary from $500 to $2,000. (At $500, we must wonder exactly how "catastrophic" the insurance is.) But the basic idea behind the MSA plans is the same. Minor health expenses are paid for by the money in an account completely at the discretion of the worker. And the worker is provided with a financial incentive to spend that money wisely. Major health expenses are covered by a high-deductible insurance. Thus, when workers are very ill, money isn't a concern.

The success of MSAs in the United States has gathered national attention. New reforms of America's big public programs for health care — Medicare for the elderly, Medicaid for the poor — have included modest roles for MSAs.

9. Can MSAs Address the Problems with Medicare?

Medical savings accounts aren't a miracle solution. But an MSA system has the potential to address many of the problems with the present health care system in Canada. Of course, the devil is in the details — a poorly designed MSA system is going to be riddled with problems. Long-term sustainability, for example, is possible with MSAs — but only if people have an incentive to spend the money in their accounts prudently and then have the ability to invest the remaining funds. But MSAs are the way to go if we're looking for an alternative that addresses medicare's woes (e.g., waiting lists, a lack of high-tech equipment, an exodus of physicians) yet preserves the characteristics we associate with an effective health care system (e.g., accessibility and timeliness).

Consider the health care experience of Crystal, a young Canadian woman with no previous health problems. Last year she experienced severe abdominal pains on an otherwise quiet May evening. The pain was still there after a week, and her family doctor suspected a gallstone attack. He called the emergency room to request that an ultrasound be performed as soon as possible to confirm the diagnosis. Crystal arrived at the hospital before 8 a.m. At 3:30 p.m., she was told that the technician had gone home and that she would have to wait until the next day for the test. Sick and feverish, she was expected to wait overnight on a gurney in the hallway of the emergency room. Finally, the following afternoon, the test was performed. Crystal had gallstones.

She was then referred to a surgeon who scheduled her for a consultation — in late July. Given the surgeon's schedule, she was lucky to have the necessary surgery within four months. Until then, Crystal could only wait. Following her doctor's orders, she changed her diet. Doing so helped, but she was still in constant pain. "People think we have the best health care system in the world," Crystal lamented to me. "They're wrong. There must be something better than this."

It's easy to understand her frustration — pain is affecting her quality of life. Crystal is simply another user of the health care system. No one within the system has a vested interest in seeing her get prompt care. The technician gets paid the same salary whether the test is performed in the late afternoon or the following morning. The hospital gets the same funding whether or not she gets the ultrasound in a timely manner. The surgeon will get the same fee whether she's operated on in November or July.

If Crystal were to pay for her own health care, matters would be different. After all, if she isn't satisfied with the service at one hospital, she can go to another one. Likewise, the surgeon's fees would be tied to her satisfaction. MSAs offer a very different approach to financing health care. Rather than the patient following the money, the money follows the patient — the difference between government funding and consumer empowerment.

Waiting lists are the biggest concern that Canadians have with their health care system. The lists are not a medical but an economic problem. Because patients have no incentive to think twice about using health care services, policy makers are forced to find ways to ration health care. Making patients wait for treatments and tests is how provincial governments have opted to ration health care.

If waiting lists develop within an MSA system, they won't be tolerated (and certainly not encouraged) but rather viewed as a bottleneck in the system. Because health care providers under such a system compete for patient funding, the bottleneck will be viewed as an opportunity — providers will have a direct financial incentive to try to address the problem, whether by hiring more nurses and technicians or by acquiring new equipment and facilities. Remember that in Canada shortages rarely occur with, say, food. At Christmas time, when consumers demand more fruitcake, bakers respond — they have a financial interest to do so. The problem with the health care system today is that no one really has this interest.

But how would physicians react to an MSA system in Canada? It's difficult to tell how much the brain drain has to do with physicians leaving for better working conditions in the United States and how much it has to do with the straight income (and tax) difference. MSAs would surely lessen the former cause — with the doctor-patient relationship restored, doctors can go back to worrying about serving patients' needs without excessive concern for provincial regulations and audits.

As for income, doctors could experiment with their billing schedules. In areas where doctors are underpaid relative to the United States, they could try to bridge the gap. Realistically, the tax difference combined with the weak performance of the Canadian dollar is significant enough that our doctors will probably be paid less under any type of system. Whether or not the federal government should address the tax issue and its effects on other sectors of the economy is beyond the scope of this book.

7.3 Final Thoughts

Many questions remain unanswered. Most arise from the vagueness of the MSA concept. What limits should be placed on an individual's ability to spend the money in a medical savings account? Should, for example, massage therapy be covered? What regulations should the government impose on health care providers? What sort of transition would be required to move to an MSA system?

These are good questions, and there are many more. But all are questions of practicality. For the moment, they are unimportant. Canadians must make a big decision first. We must decide on the direction of health care reform. Ultimately, this direction boils down to a painfully straightforward question: are we capable of making our own health care decisions?

It's a curious question. After all, in no other area do we assume that we aren't capable of rational decision making. We decide which foods to eat, where to live, which jobs to take. Such decisions affect everything from our lunchtime meals to our lifelong occupations.

But when it comes to health care, the experts believe that we are immature. Incapable of deciding when a cough is just a cold and when it's more serious. Incapable of deciding when a trip to the doctor is warranted and when it's just wasteful. Incapable of deciding if a CT scan is really necessary or whether it's just satisfying hypochondriac neurosis. This isn't to suggest that Canadians are capable of making such decisions without proper advice. We need to make informed decisions.

And, if we don't make the hard decisions, someone else will. If we are treated like fools, thought to be incapable of rational decisions, then others must act for us. Increasingly in the past few years, these decisions have been made by provincial bureaucrats.

The evidence overwhelmingly suggests that this approach isn't working. After more than a decade of health care "reform," Canadians are more concerned than ever about the quality of health care in this country. No wonder — reform has been a euphemism for greater government control over hospital administration, the ability of physicians to practise medicine, the availability of diagnostic equipment, and so on.

This book suggests that there's an alternative. Rather than further centralizing power in the hands of provincial governments, health care reform should focus on individual choice and competition. The best way to do so is to introduce medical savings accounts. Such an approach would preserve the stongest elements of medicare, but it would also address the glaring, and worsening, problems. Indeed, such a system would embody the five pillars of health care: timeliness, quality, patient orientation, cost effectiveness, and accessibility.

The transition from the present system to this new one won't be easy. The first step — and it's a big one — is that the federal government allow the provinces to experiment with health care delivery. If authoritarians in Singapore, communists in China, and profit-minded entrepreneurs in the United States all recognize the value of individual choice in health care and the potential of MSAs, why can't the Canadian federal government?

8

Real Health Care Reform in Action

IT'S DIFFICULT to remember the simplicity of ordering coffee just a decade or two ago in North America. Even the most wonderful culinary experience ended with a drab, tortured cup of coffee. The caption of an old *Punch* comic read: "Look here, if this is coffee, I want tea; but if this is tea, then I wish for coffee."

How times have changed. The big decision for coffee lovers is no longer whether or not to opt for a splash of milk. Even the local doughnut store offers cappuccino and café au lait. The corner grocery store stocks half a dozen types of beans. Enter one of the hundreds of coffee bars that have sprouted up on the landscape in recent years and choosing how to get a caffeine buzz can be difficult. Mocaccino or cappuccino? Kenyan, Ethiopian, or Indonesian? Chocolate sprinkles or cinnamon? The variety ranges from a heavy shot of espresso to the imaginative mingle of coffee and exotic flavourings.

Michael Cox, vice-president of the Federal Reserve Bank of Dallas, and Richard Alm, a business writer for the *Dallas Morning News*, argue that the trend seen in coffee — the explosion in variety and the increase in quality — applies to nearly all goods and services. In their book, *Myths of Rich and Poor*, they take a unique approach to cost comparison: the amount of work required to make a purchase. Using this comparison, they argue that prices have been falling for all goods and services, while quality has been improving. In 1954, for example, a television delivered a fuzzy picture for a big price: three months of work. Today the average American worker can get a crystal-clear picture on a 25-inch model for just three days of labour (45). A raspy three-minute call from New York to San Francisco required a whopping 90 hours of labour in 1915 (43). Today such a call, crystal clear, easily fits the budget of any family with teenage kids, costing under two minutes of work. (The figures are for American workers making American wages. Given the weak dollar and high taxes in Canada, Canadian statistics are slightly different. The basic trend, however, is the same.)

Much of *Code Blue* has focused on what's wrong with the present health care system in Canada. The previous two chapters outlined the reasons for a bold break from our "free" system and the framework within which medical savings accounts (MSAs) might be established. Based on the experiences of three generations of the Wilson family, this chapter offers a glimpse of how MSAs would actually work, moving from the abstract economic concept to everyday examples.

MSAs work well for the Wilsons — as they would for your family or mine — because they offer a financial incentive to use health care wisely. As Steven E. Landsburg notes in *The Armchair Economist: Economics and Everyday Life*, "Most of economics can be summarized in four words: 'People respond to incentives.' The rest is commentary" (3).

But this epilogue attempts to do more, describing the creative energy that would be released by medical savings accounts. If choice and competition were introduced into our health care system, the forces that have so improved our daily lives — bettering coffee, slashing the price of Internet access, and improving colour television — would transform medical services. The reasons for MSAs aren't simply born of the fire of economic necessity; they also arise for a compelling reason: to unleash creativity.

Several scenarios follow for the Wilson family. Bill, Karen, and Mary are middle-aged siblings. Wayne and Margaret, their parents, are in their late sixties. The scenarios take place in the future, after MSAs were adopted in every province beginning in 2002.

8.1 Mr. Wilson Goes to the Physician

Bill Wilson is a convert of sorts. Drop by his suburban house and he'll gleefully tell you about the merits of medical savings accounts. His best friend jokes that Bill sounds like a government ad. Bill wasn't always so keen on MSAs, though. He was fairly cynical when they were first introduced.

Before 1998, Bill never gave much thought to health care. Like many Canadians, he took it for granted that the government-run system would always be there for him. He'd heard of problems with medicare, but he dreaded any alternative. He didn't want an "American-style" system with huge medical bills every time a doctor looked in his direction.

In February 1998, Bill had an unsettling experience. When a lingering cold seemed to settle in his lungs, he just couldn't catch his breath.

His lips turned blue, and he grew faint. He was rushed to the local emergency room by ambulance. A bad chest infection, diagnosed by the doctor as pneumonia, was literally suffocating him.

At first, Bill was impressed with his care. Within an hour of arriving at the hospital, two physicians and a nurse saw him, took blood for testing, and gave him oxygen.

Then the nightmare began. Because of a bed shortage, Bill wasn't sent to a room upstairs. He spent two days in the hallway of the hospital's ER. There was no privacy. The elderly woman in the next bed was too weak to go to the restroom. Nurses gave her a bedpan, and she relieved herself in full public view.

Bill recovered completely from his bout of pneumonia. But he found the experience troubling, even humiliating. He began to wonder what would happen if he got sick again. Bill asked his wife, "Will medicare be there when we really need it?"

News about health care began to catch his eye. He discovered that problems with health care occurred all the time. In conversations with friends, Bill was struck by the number of horror stories. A man three houses down was forced to take six months off work while he waited for heart bypass surgery.

At first, Bill assumed that the problems were caused by a lack of money. Like many Canadians, he believed that health care funding had decreased during the 1990s. He thus rejoiced when the federal minister of finance introduced the "health care" budget of 1999.

And maybe it did make a small difference. With much fanfare, his provincial government hired more nurses with the extra money. But within a couple of years, the old problems had returned. His local newspaper even began running a "health care horror story" each day.

Bill didn't understand what was happening. He began reading up on health care. To his surprise, he discovered that health care spending hadn't decreased in the 1990s. In fact, spending had risen by 33% from 1990 to 1998. "Maybe it's not about money," Bill began to believe.

He thus came to the next conclusion: "It's not the amount of money, it's how the money is used." As Bill learned about the disastrous decisions his provincial government was making, he grew angry. For the first time in his life, he got involved in a political campaign — he began to work for one of the opposition parties.

But after the party was elected in 2001, not much changed. Sure, there was a new minister of health and a round of consultation, but the basic structure stayed the same.

Bill discovered that, despite the varying ideologies of the provincial governments across the country, the policies were identical when it came to health care. A young policy analyst joked that government officials were so much in synch that, "Sitting at his desk in Regina, the Saskatchewan deputy minister of health sneezes; the Ontario deputy minister of health, sitting at his desk in Toronto, says, 'Bless you.'"

Bill was also troubled by the fact that medicare's planners had such a poor track record: after more than three decades of planning and reforms, the system was a mess. In the 1980s, they closed hospital beds to "spend the money better," and waiting lists started to grow long. Then they introduced regional control and community care. And waiting lists only grew longer.

It wasn't that these changes were unreasonable. It made sense, after all, to have regional coordination of activities through some sort of health board. But these reforms did little to better the system. After all the consultations, reports, and speeches, medicare standards continued to decline. Those who ran the system had no real insight into how to fix it.

More bothersome still was Bill's discovery that insight had been lacking from day one. When medicare was first introduced, government officials forecast that by 1996 medicare would cost about $133 per person, adjusting for inflation (Levant 3). In 1996, medicare topped $2,500 per person — almost a twentyfold miscalculation.

Still, Bill assumed that if provinces focused on spending money more wisely, many of the problems could be solved. A friend was intrigued by Bill's faith in government management. "I don't doubt that money is wasted in our health care system. But has government ever managed to be efficient? What makes you think that the bureaucrats who run the CBC and Canada Post are able to make the right health care decisions?" Bill was struck by the comments. "Certainly," his friend added, "you wouldn't trust them to run your grocery store. Why do you trust them with your health care?"

Still, Bill was no fan of medical savings accounts when they were first introduced. He wondered if the changes were some sort of Americanization of the Canadian health care system. He even signed a local petition to that effect. And he had good reason to worry: how would these changes affect his children?

Alberta adopted MSAs in 2002, and Ontario soon did likewise. Many other provinces signed on. By 2007, every province had some form of an MSA.

The models differ from province to province, but all adhere to the three basic principles of medical savings accounts: people pay directly for minor health expenses — first out of their accounts, then out of their pockets; for catastrophic expenses, people are covered by a high-deductible insurance; and there is a financial incentive for people to spend wisely.

In Alberta, for example, the government requires people to put a certain minimum amount of their income into a tax-free medical savings account. The amount of money people can allocate to their accounts is flexible — they can exceed this minimum. To compensate for the re-duced take-home income, taxes were cut accordingly. Legislation also requires people to purchase a high-deductible insurance, but they have the option of choosing from a number of private-sector companies.

In Bill's province, the government puts money into the account of each person. For example, a healthy young man is given $900 regardless of his income. The government then takes back part of the money for a catastrophic insurance to cover large expenses — that is, annual health expenses that exceed $2,000.

Provinces also differ in the way that unspent money can be used. In Alberta, any money left over at the end of the year can be withdrawn and — after taxes are paid — used for any non-health-related expendi-ture. Bill's nephew put 10% of his income into his account but used under $100. At year's end, he withdrew $2,000, paid the necessary taxes, and vacationed in Europe.

In Bill's province, the rules are tighter. At retirement, money can be used for home care, personal care homes, and several other services. If an individual's account exceeds $50,000, the moneys can be withdrawn. When the individual dies, any remaining amount becomes part of the estate.

Despite his initial concerns, Bill soon discovered the attraction of the new system: MSAs empower patients by giving them health care dol-lars directly. In the United States, as in Canada before the changes, health care decisions were increasingly made by bureaucrats. With MSAs, Bill makes his own choices.

When MSAs were first introduced, provincial governments insisted that they were not about saving money but about improving the deliv-ery of health care. As Bill knew from his own reading, researchers from Queen's University and the University of Ottawa estimated in the late 1990s that $7 billion — almost 10% of total spending — could be saved if health care delivery were more efficient (Gillies). Governments tried to find ways to save money under medicare. Their efforts were always doomed to failure because the system itself was riddled with perverse incentives: for the patient, to overuse health services; for the doctor, to overprovide care; for the administrator, to defend his or her territory. MSAs, however, eliminated these perverse incentives.

And while Bill's provincial government spends roughly the same amount of money since the introduction of MSAs as before, there's a world of difference. It's like the government uses a different currency — an MSA dollar is worth so much more than a medicare dollar. The latter, after all, went straight to providers such as hospitals, which were free to spend the money as they saw fit. Sometimes they spent it wisely; sometimes they didn't. An MSA dollar goes to people, who choose how to spend it. If a hospital has many administrators and high overhead costs, its services will cost more. Patients are then tempted to go to a better-run and lower-cost hospital. A more efficient system is the result.

Because his health is good, Bill rarely sees doctors. Year after year, the money in his MSA goes unspent. In his province, as in every other province, the balance in an account at the end of a fiscal year is simply carried over into the next year's account. Bill invests a portion of his MSA in a government-approved mutual fund. His account is like a tax-free registered retirement savings plan. In the first two years of investing, Bill got a return of 12% per year.

His account is growing nicely. Given that his health is good, for the next 20 years or so, Bill will probably be able to accrue a fair amount of money. And that's important, because health care usage goes up with age. So, too, does the need for home care, personal care homes, and such services. By saving now, when he's healthy, Bill will be better able to afford these services in his elderly years.

But even for Bill, a man in good health, the new system means big changes. New services are available. For example, he pays $50 a year for the MedInformation Service, telephone access to medical information 24 hours a day, seven days a week. Instead of going to a family doctor whenever he feels unwell, he first calls MedInformation. A nurse answers his call and discusses his medical concerns.

Bill used the service a week after subscribing to it. He had developed a cough, sneezing, and a runny nose. He thought that it must be a cold — but he never got colds. Still sneezing after three days, he called

MedInformation. He discussed his symptoms with a nurse, who reassured him that he only had a cold. She then e-mailed him information on the common cold and on warning signs of a more serious condition. "If the symptoms persist after seven days," she advised, "see your doctor." The next month, he called about a rash. Again there was no need for concern. In just one month, MedInformation had paid for itself by enabling him to avoid unnecessary visits to a doctor.

But the real benefit of the MSA system is that Bill knows it will be there when he needs it — he can rely on the money in his account. Under the old system, he relied on the decisions made for him by government bureaucrats. Today he relies on his own judgement.

8.2 Chris's Health

For Karen, Bill's sister, health care isn't an issue of public policy, economics, or politics. It's personal. Chris, her son, suffers from a chronic lung disease. He was diagnosed with it as a child, and since then his illness has dominated her life: there are numerous appointments with doctors, visits to the respiratory therapist, hospital stays.

Under the old system, Karen joked with her friends, she was fighting not just her son's disease but also the system. She had good reason to be cynical. In 1997, her regional health board decided to make pediatric respiratory care "one-stop shopping." All services and diagnostic machinery were relocated to a downtown hospital. Previously, Chris was seen by a respiratory therapist once a week at a clinic a kilometre from their house. After the advent of "convenient care," Karen had to drive Chris downtown once a week.

The move also influenced his hospital care. When Chris developed a serious lung infection (a potentially life-threatening condition given that his lungs didn't work well under the best of circumstances), Karen would take him to the nearby ER. Since the pediatric respiratory specialists were moved downtown, the physicians at the ER would only assess him and begin treatment. When he was very sick, he would be admitted — to the hospital across the city. Short of breath and hacking with a cough, Chris would be sent by ambulance downtown.

The regional health board was busy changing health care for everyone. As a result, clashes between boards and physicians were common. Sometimes there were full-blown work stoppages as doctors protested funding levels or organizational decisions. Contract negotiations with the nurses' union and the support staff often resulted in strikes. Chris's care was never jeopardized, but the stoppages were a nuisance. Appointments would be cancelled, tests delayed.

Nonetheless, Karen feared the introduction of medical savings accounts. Another mother, whose child was also affected by a chronic disease, summarized her feelings when she said, "MSAs make economic sense. But our kids' illnesses aren't economic." Karen became particularly anxious when she considered that Chris could one day need a lung transplant. The expense of the procedure made her wonder if MSAs would make it impossible for Chris to get the surgery.

As it turned out, Karen had little to worry about. Recognizing the chronic nature of Chris's condition, the provincial government put him in a special health care category. As his legal decision maker, Karen receives money for his basic care (e.g., respiratory therapy and visits to doctors). If the money is exhausted, she can apply for more. All hospital expenses are covered by the government.

At first glance, then, not much seems to have changed for Chris under the MSA system. If he develops a lung infection and needs hospitalization, it isn't as though Karen has to sell her car. In fact, she never pays out of pocket. Nonetheless, much has changed. Take, for example, the home oxygen program. Because an infection compromises his ability to get enough oxygen for his body, Chris is often given oxygen-enriched air in the hospital, a standard treatment. But he doesn't need to be in the hospital every time he gets an infection. For milder bouts, a prescription of antibiotics and the home oxygen program are sufficient.

Under medicare, home oxygen was difficult to get. True, if Chris had a low blood-oxygen saturation, the government paid for oxygen tanks to be delivered to his home. But the service was available only to those who had very low oxygen saturation levels. On a couple of occasions, Chris was admitted to the hospital because his health was so poor, yet his oxygen saturation wasn't low enough to qualify him for the provincial program. Even when he did meet the criteria, the government program was slow to process his claim. If home oxygen was ordered on a Tuesday, the weekend could pass before the tanks would arrive — long days of reduced activity and long nights of sleeplessness.

For this reason, Karen stopped fussing with the provincial assistance; when Chris needed oxygen at home, she would call a private company. Within hours, the tanks would be delivered — along with a huge bill.

"It's not cheap," she once told Chris when the delivery truck arrived, "but we have the money." Karen quietly recognized that in many ways Canada had a two-tiered health care system. For the moment, she could afford better care for her son.

With medical savings accounts, these worries are gone. When Chris needs oxygen at home, Karen picks up the phone and orders it. There are no provincial forms to fill out, and she doesn't have to reach for her chequebook. Because the government gives them money to contract such services directly, they are free to do so when necessary. The province, after all, doesn't provide the service; rather, it empowers patients (or their legal guardians) to contract the service, and home oxygen supply has become a competitive business. Numerous companies compete for contracts, and prices have fallen.

The system isn't perfect. Because Chris is categorized as "chronically ill," Karen doesn't have the freedom with his medical savings account that she has with her own. There are more restrictions and an annual audit. But labour disruptions don't interfere with his care any longer. And, with a clinic specializing in respiratory care opening in the neighbourhood, the weekly trip downtown for therapy will soon end.

8.3 Mary and the Migraine

"There you go again," jokes Mary Wilson each time her brother carries on about medical savings accounts. Mary, who turned 42 last month, doesn't follow politics or political issues. Unlike Bill, who spends hours reading about health care, she hasn't given much thought to the issue.

Mary may not be able to rattle off the latest statistics on Singapore's experiment with medical savings accounts, but she does know everything about her own MSA. She can tell you exactly how much money she has in her account. No wonder — she manages her finances carefully. She regards the dollars in her MSA as her own.

Under medicare, Mary didn't even have a family doctor. If she became ill, she usually drove to the nearest walk-in clinic. When it was closed, or if the lineup was too long, she'd go to a hospital ER. Once she went to the ER with a sore throat. After running some tests, the physician impatiently asked, "Exactly why are you here? You could see your family doctor in the morning."

"Why should I wait?" Mary replied.

Mary doesn't go to the emergency room for a sore throat anymore;

if she did, she'd receive a bill for $125. True, every year she has over $700
put into her account after paying for catastrophic insurance, but why
waste it? The family doctor up the street will see her for $20.

Last year, Mary learned the real value of her MSA. One afternoon at
work, she developed a severe headache and had to go home. At first,
she thought nothing of it. But when she experienced a similar headache the next month, she became concerned. Her secretary suggested
that they may be migraines.

Mary booked an appointment with her family physician for the next
morning. After giving her a quick examination, he explained that the
pain could well be due to a migraine. They discussed her options: she
could have a CT scan or an MRI scan to rule out anything more serious. Mary opted for the CT scan. The MRI scan was overkill and expensive. A CT scan would do. She probably didn't need a test, but why
take a chance? After all, she had enough money in her MSA.

Under medicare, CT scans weren't easy to get. True, the waiting lists
were nothing compared with those for MRI scans. But waiting was
very much a part of the diagnostic process. Because medicare carried
no direct costs for patients, they never hesitated to get tests. Provincial
governments therefore had to find a way to save money, and they allowed lengthy waiting lists to develop for basic diagnostic tests.

When a colleague from work described how long she'd had to wait
for a breast biopsy, Mary was reminded of the stories her cousins told
about their early life in the Soviet Union and how they used to line up
for toilet paper. Government rationing isn't a Canadian phenomenon.
It happens wherever governments hold a monopoly on goods and services and attempt to contain costs.

With MSAs, though, governments don't need to ration care. People
are responsible, within limits, for the financial consequences of their
health care decisions.

CT scanners used to be found only in hospitals. But after the introduction of medical savings accounts, private companies began to buy
the equipment and offer the service to patients. After all, patient demand exceeded the supply provided by the handful of hospital scanners. And these private companies offered the newest technology.
Unlike the antique models that hospitals typically owned, private CT
scanners are top of the line.

Providing diagnostic services such as CT scans is a cutthroat business. There are no government grants — like any business, providers

must offer their services at competitive rates. Otherwise, people will spend their MSA dollars elsewhere. Prices have dropped dramatically in recent years. In Mary's hometown, it's now possible to have a CT scan within an hour, complete with a reading by a certified radiologist.

So, after talking to her physician, Mary started to call around. One company wanted $500 for the scan. She thought that was a bit high. After making some more calls, she finally found a facility that could book her first thing in the morning. The price was right: $395 plus taxes. This type of cost-conscious shopping would never have taken place under medicare.

Today Mary views health care as another basic need — like housing, clothing, or food. And, like finding a better apartment to live in, buying a new winter jacket, or shopping for the week's groceries, she looks for the best value for her dollar.

And it's not just getting a CT scan that's so different. With the introduction of MSAs, the doctor-patient relationship has been reestablished. Doctors no longer serve the provincial billing schedule; they now serve patients. Primary care has thus been revolutionized.

Some doctors, for instance, reject the very idea of a basic fee schedule. Dr. Duane Funk, who served as president of the Canadian Medical Association, champions this view: "How can you say that a physical exam is worth $10 or $15 or $20? Everyone is different. Everyone has different concerns. Some people require more time, others less." For this reason, he charges an hourly rate in his practice. His patients, as a result, never feel rushed. Other physicians have also experimented with billing.

Some physicians have banded together and formed 24-hour clinics. Others ensure all-day and all-night care for their patients by guaranteeing a doctor on call. These clinics tend to charge slightly more for their services. In selecting family physicians, people can look around and pick whom they want.

In many ways, medical services are like any other service. There are hundreds of ideas about how they should be offered. And every consumer-patient has different preferences. When provincial governments ran the health care system, however, there was only one basic way to offer health care services, because there was only one basic billing schedule. Today that's all changed.

Perhaps those who have benefited most from the surge in creative energy are the chronically ill. Recognizing this niche, physicians established specialized clinics, often working with nurses and physiothera-

pists. In Mary's city, there are hundreds of such clinics now — for patients who suffer from diabetes, depression, breast cancer, or some
other disease. One such clinic serves her 67-year-old father, Wayne,
very well.

8.4 Preventing the Complications of Wayne's Diabetes

Ten years ago, Wayne didn't react well to the news that he had non-
insulin-dependent diabetes. "Diabetes!" he said to his physician. "Are
you crazy?" Up to that point in his life, health had never been a problem. How could he have diabetes?

At first, he ignored the doctor's diagnosis. "There must have been a
mistake with the diagnosis," he reasoned. He didn't return any of the
calls from the doctor's office for two weeks.

Eventually, though, Wayne came around. He began to watch what
he ate more carefully. Still, blood-glucose control was a problem. At
some level, he just didn't accept his illness.

Maybe it was the introduction of MSAs, or the endless nagging of
his daughter, but Wayne eventually changed his ways. MSAs, after all,
hold people accountable for their health care decisions. Wayne knew full
well that if he didn't control his blood sugar, he would run into problems. The money he'd want to withdraw from his account wouldn't be
there. Instead, it would have been spent on medical bills.

Two years ago, a hormone specialist opened a clinic with several
family physicians for people with diabetes. For a flat yearly fee, Wayne
subscribes to their "Diabetica A" program. As part of the package, he
sees a family physician every three months to discuss the control of his
blood sugar. Medications are sometimes adjusted during these sessions,
and sometimes tests are run to determine the progress of his disease
(tests that look for protein in the urine, changes in vision, etc.).

Wayne also has regular meetings with the clinic's dietitian. The
nurse is always available to answer questions about his condition.
When he first subscribed to the service, she provided tips on "eating
with diabetes." And every three weeks a nurse comes to his house and
trims his toenails. Foot care for a diabetic is important — one of the
most common reasons for hospitalization is infection of the foot.

This service isn't cheap, but Wayne thinks it's worthwhile. There is,
then, a perfect exchange: for the clinic, Wayne provides revenue; for
Wayne, the clinic provides a useful service.

8.5 Margaret's Vision Problems

Margaret married Wayne nearly 45 years ago. They have been blessed with three healthy children and a peaceful existence.

Like many aging couples, Wayne and Margaret have their share of health problems. Margaret was diagnosed with the early stages of osteoporosis last March.

The big scare for Margaret, however, was something she hadn't mentioned even to her husband: she was going blind, or so she thought. At first, the problem seemed minor. Stop signs began to blur when she drove around the city.

Eventually, Margaret booked an appointment with her family physician. It took the doctor less than a minute to figure out the problem. She had a cataract in her left eye. The condition was not only benign but also reversible. Given the problems her decrease in vision posed, he suggested that she consider cataract surgery.

Choosing where to get such surgery requires far more effort than the decision to get it. After the MSA health reforms, cataract clinics opened up around the city. The surgery, after all, is fairly minor. There's no need for the high overhead cost of a hospital. So eye surgeons set up private clinics offering a variety of services.

After the diagnosis, Margaret phoned around and found several clinics to her liking. To her surprise, each one offered her a tour. She started with the one closest to her home, the VisionCare Clinic. A nurse showed her around, pointing out the latest equipment acquired by the clinic. Margaret was particularly impressed with the clinic's efforts to reduce the rates of infection. The operating theatres, for example, have slightly higher air pressure than the other rooms. As a result, when the OR doors are opened, air (and the bacteria swimming in it) don't rush in. The tour closed with a lengthy discussion about the standards of care. VisionCare not only meets provincial regulations and national standards but also scores well in the annual national survey of a well-respected health care magazine. Margaret visited the other clinics but eventually decided on VisionCare.

To her, there's something marvellous about the process. Health care is no longer a giant black box. In the late 1990s, for instance, her cousin had a brush with breast cancer, diagnosed after a lump was taken out of her left breast. Her oncologist suggested radiation therapy and slated her for the treatment at the local hospital. But what assurances did she have that the machine worked properly? If she became sicker and required admission to a hospital, what did she ultimately know about that hospital?

At the time, Margaret was struck by the irony: getting proper health care is a life-and-death decision, whereas buying a dishwasher is hardly that significant. Yet it was easier for her cousin to find out about consumer satisfaction with a Maytag than the effectiveness of cancer care at the local hospital.

In a government-run system, providers of health care had little reason to be accountable. Sure, some groups of hospitals occasionally published surveys, but the information was of little use. Under the MSA system, there's a competitive market for providers, thereby pushing them to be accountable and to meet high standards. And there's a competitive market for health information. Bookstores stock numerous consumer guides, from a Canadian version of *America's Best Hospitals* to *The Consumer Guide to Coronary Artery Bypass Graft Surgery*. Magazines advise patients on "how to get the best bang for the MSA buck" and "101 ways to improve your health without breaking your MSA." Web sites boasting "the most comprehensive reviews of radiation therapy" and "clinics of excellence" have been posted by consumers' groups, physicians' committees, and patients' advocates.

*   *   *

The ideas outlined in this chapter may seem more like fiction than public policy. An end to waiting lists? Competition between providers? More health information? It sounds so remarkably different from the present system. And it is.

The biggest public policy issue Canada will face in the next century is health care. The roads diverge. Canadians must choose between a government-run monolith or a system run by the people who use it. About the latter approach, *National Post* columnist Andrew Coyne recently wrote that

> The task will be to import market mechanisms within the envelope of public finance, allowing choice and competition free reign while preserving universal coverage and equality of access. These "social markets" will usefully blur the line between public and private, revealing the true justification of markets: not vehicles for private enrichment, but for harnessing of private interests to the public good.

Medical savings accounts offer a way of doing just that.

Notes

CHAPTER 1

1. Data taken from Statistics Canada's Public Use Microdata File, General Social Survey — Health, 1991.

2. For the purposes of its analysis, the Fraser Institute classified cardiovascular surgery into three groups in order of priority: emergent, urgent, and elective. This division is based on the work of Dr. C. David Naylor and his associates. See Naylor et al.

3. For such analysis, data were not simply drawn from the survey but also provided by the University of Alberta Hospitals, Saskatchewan Health, the Manitoba Cardiac Sciences Program, the Newfoundland and Labrador Department of Health and Community Services, and the Montreal Regional Health Board.

4. The waiting times for radiotherapy in the Mackillop study are similar to those found by the Fraser Institute study. *Waiting Your Turn* underestimated the waiting lists for prostate cancer patients.

5. Medical students are required to have an undergraduate degree. Assuming that a student only gets a general science degree (rather than a full four-year degree) and then does the regular four-year medical degree plus the two years of additional training to become a family physician, the costs are enormous. According to the *University of Manitoba Institutional Analysis Book 1994–95*, a year in science costs the taxpayer about $3,000, and medical studies are closer to $25,000. The math is straightforward: 3 x $3,000 + 6 x $25,000 = $159,000.

CHAPTER 3

1. For example, with capital costs, they observe that hospitals do take into account greater depreciation to a larger extent than Krasny and Ferrier have probably assumed (160).

2. Percent GDP = 100% x total health care expenditures / GDP.

3. Another major study on the uninsured was conducted recently by the Employee Benefit Research Institute. The study found that over a 12-month period, from October 1994 to September 1995, 7.4% of nonelderly Americans had no insurance (see Copeland 1).

4. In 1987, employers provided health care coverage to 69% of the nonelderly population. By 1993, the level had dropped to 64%, where it remains today. Small businesses seem to be the most inclined not to provide health insurance to employees.

According to a Dun and Bradstreet survey, in 1998 only 39% offered coverage; just two years earlier, 46% of small businesses offered such coverage (see Bernstein; and Koretz).

5. An extensive American study that looked at seven and a half years of media coverage, examining over 2,100 randomly selected stories, concluded that most media coverage was neutral in overall tone. "However, the tone of coverage has become more critical over time and differs dramatically by source of media. The most visible media sources — television and newspaper special series — conveyed negative stories in more than half of their coverage and most often used anecdotes in telling their stories" (Brodie, Brady, and Altman 10).

6. In his speech, Walker noted that the insurance companies do compete with each other and thus provide consumer choice. "We already have managed care," he said, "what we need is competition."

CHAPTER 4

1. *Achieving Health for All: A Framework for Health Promotion* (Canada, 1986), *The Report of the Ontario Panel on Health Goals* (Ontario, 1987), *Report of Ontario Health Review Panel* (Ontario, 1987), *Report of the Commission of Inquiry into Health and Social Services* (Quebec, 1988), *Report of the Commission on Selected Health Care Programs* (New Brunswick, 1989), *Future Directions for Health Care in Saskatchewan: Report of the Saskatchewan Commission on Directions in Health Care* (Saskatchewan, 1990), *The Report of the Nova Scotia Royal Commission on Health Care* (Nova Scotia, 1990), *The Rainbow Report: Our Vision of Health, Report of the Premier's Commission on Health Care for Albertans* (Alberta, 1990), *Report of the British Columbia Commission on Health Care and Costs* (British Columbia, 1991), *The First Report of the Standing Committee on Health and Welfare, Social Affairs, Seniors, and the Status of Women* (Canada, 1991), *The Report of the Prince Edward Island Task Force on Health* (Prince Edward Island, 1992), *Quality Health for Manitobans: The Action Plan* (Manitoba, 1992), and *Report on the Reduction of Hospital Services* (Newfoundland, 1993).

2. Most Canadian experts are adamantly opposed to user fees and have written frequently on the topic. The now-defunct Ontario Premier's Council on Health, Well-Being, and Social Justice, for example, published seven reports on the topic, including *The Remarkable Tenacity of User Charges* (see Barer et al.) and *User Charges in Health Care: A Bibliography* (see Evans et al.).

3. For a discussion of these studies, see Ramsay, "Medical" 22–23.

4. There were three user-fee groups. The statistics quoted compare the free-care group with the 95% user-fee group. For more information, see Newhouse and the Insurance Experiment Group parts 2 and 3.

5. It's not necessarily true that all of these options are still available to patients in every province. Direct access to specialists, for example, is increasingly limited. The point is that in a free system the incentive to overconsume naturally leads a patient to demand the highest-trained physician without regard for the seriousness of the ailment.

6. A similar point, with many examples, is made in chapter 4 of Rachlis and Kushner, *Strong Medicine*.

7. See Priest, *Operating in the Dark*.
8. Local descriptions of the emergency room crises ran in dailies such as the *Winnipeg Free Press*, the *Toronto Sun*, and the Montreal *Gazette*. For good summaries of the events, see Coutts, "Why"; Gratzer, "Guest Column"; and Sillars.

CHAPTER 6

1. There are, of course, areas in which Decter refuses to recognize medicare's deficiencies. As noted earlier, his analysis of waiting lists (e.g., "Often patients wish to have surgery scheduled some time in the future" [209]) is innocently naïve at best, calculatingly manipulative at worst.
2. Adapted from a similar analysis of the American health care sector. See Goodman and Musgrave 20.
3. See, e.g., Boyer 27–29. He intelligently argues in favour of user fees for three full pages but never considers how such a policy would be implemented.
4. Claude Forget, a former Quebec minister of health, coauthored a book advocating internal markets for Canada with his wife, Monique Jerome-Forget, a former federal assistant deputy minister of health and welfare. Their model is slightly different from the structure mentioned here, but the problems that arise from their proposed reforms are similar to those of the British-style reforms and are outlined in the next section. See Forget and Jerome-Forget.
5. Prime Minister Tony Blair announced reforms in 1998 that limit these financial perks within the NHS.
6. Borrowed from an analogy on higher education in Frum, *Dead Right* 191.

CHAPTER 7

1. In fact, Singapore's demographics are comparable to Canada's. In 1990, 8.5% of the population in Singapore was over the age of 60. By 2030, 29.4% of the population is projected to be over 60 (Asher 2).

Works Cited

Abraham, Carolyn. "Canadian Doctors Take Their Talents South." *Globe and Mail* 11 July 1998: A1.

Abraham, Carolyn, and Sean Fine. "Patients Must Wait for Care." *Globe and Mail* 25 July 1998: A6.

"American Opinion." *Wall Street Journal* 25 June 1998: A9–14.

Angus Reid Group. "As Parliament Re-Opens, Healthcare and Liberals Hand-in-Hand as Chart Leaders." Press release. 1 Feb. 1999.

Armstrong, Jack. Telephone interview. Dec. 1996.

Armstrong, Pat, and Hugh Armstrong. *Universal Health Care: What the United States Can Learn from the Canadian Experience.* New York: New, 1998.

——. *Wasting Away: The Undermining of Canadian Health Care.* Toronto: Oxford UP, 1996.

Arnett, Grace-Marie, and Melindia Schriver. "State Lessons in Health Regulations." *Washington Times* 24 July 1998: A19.

Arnett, Jr., Jerome C. "Ontario's Health Care: A Pox on Doctors and Patients." *Wall Street Journal* 12 July 1996: A13.

"As Health System Shrinks, Elderly Slip off the Edges." *Toronto Star* 23 Sept. 1995: A16.

Asher, Mukul G. "Compulsory Savings in Singapore: An Alternative to the Welfare State." National Center for Policy Analysis, Dallas, TX, Policy Report 198, 1995.

Barchet, Stephen. *Medical Savings Accounts: A Building Block for Sound Health Care.* Seattle: Evergreen Freedom Foundation, 1995.

Barer, Morris L., and Robert G. Evans. "Interpreting Canada: Models, Mind-Sets, and Myths." *Health Affairs* 11.1 (1992): 44–61.

Barnett, Vicki. "Bilingualism, Medicare on Reform List." *Calgary Herald* 15 Aug. 1988: B1.

Baxter, David, and Andrew Rambo. *Healthy Choices: Demographics and Health Spending in Canada, 1980 to 2035.* Vancouver: Urban Futures Institute, 1996.

Belien, Paul. "Patient Empowerment in Europe." *Fraser Forum* Feb. 1998: 12–18.

Bell, C.M., et al. "Shopping Around for Hospital Services: A Comparison of the United States and Canada." *JAMA* 279 (1998): 1015–17.

Benk, V., et al. "Predictors of Delay in Starting Radiation Treatment for Patients with Early Stage Breast Cancer." *International Journal of Radiation Oncology, Biology, and Physics* 41.1 (1998): 109–15.

Bernstein, Aaron. "The Health Care Net Is Shrinking." *Business Week* 12 Oct. 1998: 144.

Black, Charlyn, and Noralou P. Roos. "Conventional Wisdom Not Enough." *Winnipeg Free Press* 17 Sept. 1998: A13.

Blevins, Sue. Telephone interview. May 1998.

Blomqvist, Ake. *The Health Care Business: International Evidence on Private Versus Public Health Care Systems.* Vancouver: Fraser Institute, 1979.

Bohuslawsky, Maria. "Patient Overdose: 67 a Day." *Ottawa Citizen* 24 Mar. 1998: A1.

——. "Politicians Jump Medicare Queue." *Ottawa Citizen* 6 June 1998: A1.

Borsellino, Matt. "Conference Uncovers Myths behind Surgery Waiting Lists." *Medical Post* 30 June 1998: 29.

Boyer, Patrick. *Hands-On Democracy: How You Can Take Part in Canada's Renewal.* Toronto: Stoddart, 1993.

"Brain Cramps." *Ottawa Citizen* 19 Nov. 1998: A15.

Brodie, Mollyann, Lee Ann Brady, and Drew E. Altman. "Media Coverage of Managed Care: Is There a Negative Bias?" *Health Affairs* 17.1 (1998): 9–25.

Canadian Medical Association. *1998 Physician Resource Questionnaire.* Ottawa: CMA, 1998.

Carney, Pat. "Wanted: Access to an Effective Medicare System." *Globe and Mail* 2 June 1997: A19.

Cavers, William. Telephone interview. Jan. 1999.

Chwialkowska, Luiza. "Health-Care Queue-Jumping 'A Fact of Life.'" *Ottawa Citizen* 7 June 1998: A3.

Clemens, Jason, and Cynthia Ramsay. "Health Care Isn't Free — Even in Canada." *Fraser Forum* July 1996: 5–7.

Copeland, Craig. "Characteristics of the Non-Elderly with Selected Sources of Health Insurance and Lengths of Uninsured Spells." Employee Benefit Research Institute, Washington, DC, Issue Brief 198, June 1998.

Coutts, Jane. "Cataract Delays Linked to Doctors." *Globe and Mail* 11 Aug. 1998: A3.

——. "Group Finds Support in Poll for Health Allowances Idea." *Globe and Mail* 13 Nov. 1997: A16.

——. "Patients Waiting Longer, Canadian Doctors Say." *Globe and Mail* 12 Aug. 1998: A7.

——. "Why Emergency Wards Are on the Sick List." *Globe and Mail* 27 Feb. 1998: A1.

Cox, W. Michael, and Richard Alm. *Myths of Rich and Poor: Why We're Better Off than We Think.* New York: Basic, 1999.

Crichton, Anne, et al. *Health Care: A Community Concern?* Calgary: U of Calgary P, 1997.

Currie, R.J. "The Surgical Waiting Game." *Winnipeg Free Press* 11 Aug. 1998: A13.

Daly, Rita. "Why Cancer Patients Must Wait." *Toronto Star* 7 Feb. 1999: A1.

Day, Brian. Telephone interview. Dec. 1998.

——. "The Role of Private Hospitals in a Public System." Address at the conference Putting Patients First, Toronto, 3 Nov. 1997.

Deber, Raisa. "Wrong Answers at the Wrong Time?" *Canadian Medical Association Journal* 157 (1997): 1726–27.

Deber, Raisa B., Sharmila L. Mhatre, and G. Ross Baker. "A Review of Provincial Initiatives." *Limits to Care: Reforming Canada's Health System in an Age of Restraint.* Ed. Ake Blomqvist and David M. Brown. Toronto: C.D. Howe Institute, 1994. 91–124.

De Coster, Carolyn, et al. "Surgical Waiting Times in Manitoba." Unpublished essay, Manitoba Centre for Health Policy and Evaluation, Winnipeg, 1998.

Decter, Michael B. *Healing Medicare: Managing Health System Change the Canadian Way.* Toronto: McGilligan, 1994.

DeMont, John. "Frustration in Ottawa." *Maclean's* 2 Dec. 1996: 62–64.

DePalma, Anthony. "Doctor, What's the Prognosis? A Crisis in Canada." *New York Times* 18 Dec. 1996: 3.

Dingwall, David. Speech to the House of Commons Standing Committee on Health, 30 Apr. 1996.

Dueckert, Dennis. "Medicare System Can't Survive, MDs Told." *Gazette* [Montreal] 16 Aug. 1995: A9.

Dyck, Frank J., et al. "Effect of Surveillance on the Number of Hysterectomies in the Province of Saskatchewan." *New England Journal of Medicine* 117 (1977): 1326–28.

"Emergency Overload." Editorial. *Gazette* [Montreal] 5 Feb. 1998: B2.

Enterline, Philip E., et al. "The Distribution of Medical Services before and after 'Free' Medical Care — The Quebec Experience." *New England Journal of Medicine* 289 (1973): 1174–78.

——. "Effects of 'Free' Medical Care on Medical Practice — The Quebec Experience." *New England Journal of Medicine* 288 (1973): 1152–55.

Evans, Robert G. *Strained Mercy: The Economics of Canadian Health Care.* Toronto: Butterworth, 1984.

Evans, Robert G., E.M.A. Parish, and Floyd Scully. "Medical Productivity, Scale Effects, and Demand Generation." *Canadian Journal of Economics* 6.3 (1973): 376–89.

Evans, Robert, and Noralou P. Roos. "Let's Consider What's Right about the Canadian Health Care System." *Toronto Star* 21 Sept. 1998: A11.

Ferguson, Derek. "Here's What Reformers Have Said on Health Care." *Toronto Star* 28 May 1997: A14.

Ferrara, Peter J. "More than a Theory: Medical Savings Accounts at Work." Cato Institute, Washington, DC, Policy Analysis 220, 14 Mar. 1995.

——. "A New Prescription." *Wilson Quarterly* 20.3 (1996): 25–27.

Feschuk, Scott. "Health Ministers Clash on Clinics." *Globe and Mail* 30 May 1995: A9.

Fine, Sean. "Cultures of Care." *Globe and Mail* 9 July 1998: A9.

Flanagan, Tom. Telephone interview. May 1998.

Foot, David K., with Daniel Stoffman. *Boom, Bust, and Echo: How to Profit from the Coming Demographic Shift.* Toronto: Macfarlane, 1996.

Forget, Claude, and Monique Jérôme-Forget. *Who Is the Master? A Blueprint for Canadian Health Care Reform.* Montreal: Institute for Research on Public Policy, 1998.

Fox, George A., Jonathon O'Dea, and Patrick S. Parfrey. "Coronary Artery Bypass Graft Surgery in Newfoundland and Labrador." *Canadian Medical Association Journal* 158 (1998): 1137–42.

Francis, Diane. "Ottawa Sits by as Quebec's Health Care Tab Continues to Rise." *Financial Post* 16 June 1998: 19.

——. "Random Facts and Figures from the World Economic Forum." *Financial Post* 7 Feb. 1998: 19.

Friedman, David. *Hidden Order: The Economics of Everyday Life.* New York: HarperBusiness, 1996.

Frum, David. *Dead Right.* New York: Basic, 1994.

——. "Reform and Tory Medicare Pledges Are Deceptive." *Financial Post* 17 May 1997: 22.

——. *What's Right: The New Conservatism and What It Means for Canada.* Toronto: Random, 1996.

Fuchs, Victor R. *Who Shall Live?* New York: Basic, 1974.

Gadd, Jane. "Psychiatric Shortage Blamed for Long Waits." *Globe and Mail* 3 June 1998: A2.

Gagnon, Louise. "One-Third of Hospital Days 'Inappropriate.'" *Medical Post* 7 Apr. 1998: 79.

Gavora, Carrie J. "Congress's Wrong Prescription for the HMO Headache." Heritage Foundation Backgrounder 1205, 21 July 1998.

Gawande, Atul. "Of Course You Don't Like Your HMO." *Slate* 24 Oct. 1997: 22.

Gennser, Margit. "Sweden's Health Care System." Ramsay, McArthur, and Walker 53–62.

Gillies, James. "The Case for a Health-Care Debit Card." *Globe and Mail* 27 Feb. 1999: D3.

Gillis, Charlie. "Canadians Support Private Health Care." *National Post* 22 Feb. 1999: A1.

Globerman, Steven, and Aidan Vining. *Cure or Disease? Private Health Insurance in Canada*. Toronto: U of Toronto P, 1996.

Goodman, John C., and Gerald L. Musgrave. *Patient Power: Solving America's Health Care Crisis*. Washington, DC: Cato Institute, 1992.

Goodman, William E. "Canada's Health-Care System: You Get What You Pay For." *Private Practice* Oct. 1989: 12.

Gould, David. Telephone interview. 1998.

Government of Manitoba. *Quality of Health for Manitobans: The Action Plan*. Winnipeg: Government of Manitoba, 1992.

Gratzer, David. "Canadian and US Health Care Systems Have Same Ailment." *Financial Post* 12 June 1997: 17.

——. "Guest Column: No Amount of Effort or Money Will Save Our Soviet Medicare System." *Alberta Report* 23 Mar. 1998: 37.

Gray, Charlotte. "Health Care among Forgotten Issues in Forgettable Federal Election." *Canadian Medical Association Journal* 157 (1997): 57–58.

——. "NHS Reforms Reduce Waiting Lists but Create Widespread Unease." *Canadian Medical Association Journal* 155 (1996): 1487–88.

Greenspon, Edward. "Chrétien Hazy on Drug Costs." *Globe and Mail* 7 May 1997: A1.

——. "Health Care Woes Deemed Provinces' Fault, Poll Reveals." *Globe and Mail* 6 Feb. 1999: A10.

Harper, Stephen. Telephone interview. June 1998.

Harris, Robert. Telephone interview. Aug. 1998.

The Health Services Utilization Working Group. "When Less Is Better: Using Canada's Hospitals Efficiently." Unpublished essay, 1994.

Heinrich, Jeff. "Health Care Envy of US, Kennedy Says." *Gazette* [Montreal] 19 Mar. 1996: A5.

Henderson, David. "Demand." *The Fortune Encyclopedia of Economics*. New York: Warner, 1993.

Henton, Darcy. "Patients Tell Agonizing Tales of Fallout from Hospital Cuts." *Toronto Star* 24 Sept. 1995: A18.

Hickson, G.B., W.A. Altemeier, and J.M. Perrin. "Physician Reimbursement by Salary or Fee-for-Service: Effect on Physician Practice Behaviour in a Randomized Prospective Study." *Pediatrics* 80 (1987): 344–50.

Hill, Grant. "The Health-Care Debate: One Tier or Two? What Canada's Health System Needs Is More Choice." *Globe and Mail* 21 Aug. 1995: A11.

Holle, Peter. "Notes from the Frontier: Relieving the Pressure." Unpublished essay, Frontier Centre for Public Policy, Winnipeg, 6 Apr. 1998.

Houston, Paul. "Sizable Group of Democrats Pushing 'Single-Payer' Health Plan." *Los Angeles Times* 9 Oct. 1993: A-18.

Hsiao, William C. "Medical Savings Accounts: Lessons from Singapore." *Health Affairs* 14.2 (1995): 260–66.

Hunt, Albert R. "Politicians Risk Voter Backlash This Autumn if They Ignore Call for Action." *Wall Street Journal* 25 June 1998: A9.

Institute for Clinical Evaluative Sciences. "Survey Indicates Preferential Access to Some Cardiovascular Procedures." Press release. 30 Sept. 1998.

Jensen, Gail A., and Michael A. Morrisey. "The Premium Consequences of Group Health Insurance Provisions." Unpublished essay, 1998.

Joint Advisory Committee of the Government of Ontario and the Ontario Medical Association. "Report on Methods to Control Health Care Costs." Unpublished essay, 1977.

Jones, Deborah. "His Own Private Hospital." *Canadian Medical Association Journal* 157 (1997): 297–300.

Kennedy, Mark. "Critical Condition." *Gazette* [Montreal] 13 Feb. 1999: B1.

——. "Liberals Won't Share Medicare Power." *Ottawa Citizen* 13 June 1997: A4.

Kennedy, Mark, and Francine Dube. "Canadians Want More Private Health Care: Poll." *National Post* 5 Dec. 1998: A1.

Kollek, Daniel. "Don't Blame the Hospitals for the Emergency-Room Logjam." *Globe and Mail* 10 Feb. 1998: A21.

Koop, C. Everett, et al. "Beyond Health Promotion: Reducing the Need and Demand for Medical Care." *Health Affairs* 17.2 (1998): 70–84.

Korcok, Milan. "Excess Demand Meets Excess Supply as Referral Companies Link Canadian Patients, US Hospitals." *Canadian Medical Association Journal* 157 (1997): 767–70.

——. "The Lost Generation: Flood Doors Open as Large Numbers of Canadian FPs Head South." *Canadian Medical Association Journal* 154 (1996): 893–96.

Koretz, Gene. "The Widening Health Care Gap." *Business Week* 12 Oct. 1998: 28.

Krasney, Jacques, and Ian R. Ferrier. "A Closer Look at Health Care in Canada." *Health Affairs* 10.2 (1991): 152–58.

Landsburg, Steven E. *The Armchair Economist: Economics and Everyday Life.* New York: Basic, 1993.

Lantos, Gabor. Response to a letter by Dr. Gordon. *Canadian Medical Association Journal* 154 (1996): 630.

Lem, Sharon. "Delaying Surgery a Danger." *Toronto Sun* 28 Sept. 1998: 22.

Levant, Ezra. *Youthquake.* Vancouver: Fraser Institute, 1996.

Liberal Party of Canada. *Securing Our Future Together.* Ottawa: Liberal Party of Canada, 1997.

Lifeso, Robert. Telephone interview. Aug. 1998.

"Looking toward Tomorrow: Health, Health Care, and Medicine in a Mercurial World." Unpublished essay, Canadian Medical Association, Ottawa, 1998.

Lurie, N., et al. "Termination from Medi-Cal: Does It Affect Health?" *New England Journal of Medicine* 311 (1984): 480–84.

——. "Termination from Medi-Cal Benefits: A Follow-Up Study One Year Later." *New England Journal of Medicine* 314 (1986): 1266–68.

Mackillop, W.J., Y. Zhou, and C.F. Quirt. "A Comparison of Delays in the Treatment of Cancer with Radiation in Canada and the United States." *International Journal of Radiation Oncology, Biology, and Physics* 32 (1995): 531–39.

Manning, Preston. "Health Care Reform for Canada." Speech to the 1994 Ontario Hospital Association Convention and Exhibition, 8 Nov. 1994.

——. "Out of Control Government Spending Killing Medicare." Pamphlet, Reform Party of Canada, 29 Mar. 1993.

McArthur, Keith. "What Price High-Tech Health Care?" *Winnipeg Free Press* 14 Apr. 1998: A9.

McCarthy, Shawn. "Health-System Cuts Create Two-Tier Care, Opposition Charges." *Globe and Mail* 18 Feb. 1999: A4.

McDonald, Paul, et al. *Waiting Lists and Waiting Times for Health Care in Canada: More Management!! More Money??* Ottawa: Health Canada, 1998.

Menzies, Peter. "MPs Lock Horns over Medicare Future: Manning's Proposal for Two-Tiered Scheme Termed Dangerous by Alberta Premier." *Calgary Herald* 28 Apr. 1995: A3.

Moulton, Donalee. "Bladder Cancer Survival Affected by Long Canadian Waiting Lists." *Medical Post* 21 July 1998: 5.

Mueller, Dennis C. *Public Choice II*. Cambridge: Cambridge UP, 1989.

Murley, Reginald, ed. *Patients or Customers: Are the NHS Reforms Working?* London, Eng.: Institute of Economic Affairs, 1995.

Nairne, Doug. "Crisis Creates Suicide Surge." *Winnipeg Free Press* 15 Apr. 1998: 1.

——. "Sleep Patient Tired of Waiting List." *Winnipeg Free Press* 19 June 1998: A4.

National Cancer Institute of Canada. *Canadian Cancer Statistics 1999*. Toronto: NCIC, 1999.

National Centre for Policy Analysis. *Congressional Health Care Briefing Book*. Dallas: NCPA, 1995.

The National Forum on Health. *Canada Health Action: Building on the Legacy*. Final Report. Vol. 1. Ottawa: Minister of Public Works and Government Services, 1997. 2 vols.

Naylor, C. David, et al. "Assigning Priority to Patients Requiring Coronary Revascularization: Consensus Principles from a Panel of Cardiologists and Cardiac Surgeons." *Canadian Journal of Cardiology* 7.5 (1991): 207–13.

Newhouse, Joseph P., and the Insurance Experiment Group. *Free for All? Lessons from the RAND Health Insurance Experiment*. Cambridge: Harvard UP, 1993.

"The Next Five Years." Unpublished essay, Institute for Research in Public Policy, Montreal, Policy Options 20.1, 1999.

Noseworthy, Tom. "National Forum." *The National*. CBC Television. 4 Feb. 1997.

"OMA Criticized for 'Silence' on Social Issues." *Toronto Star* 1 Dec. 1996: A12.

Ontario Task Force on the Use and Provision of Medical Services. *1989–90 Annual Report*. Toronto: Ontario Ministry of Health, 1990.

Organization for Economic Cooperation and Development. *Internal Markets in the Making: Health Systems in Canada, Iceland, and the United Kingdom.* Paris: OECD, 1995.

Organization for Economic Cooperation and Development Health Data. CD-ROM 3.6, May 1995.

Pagtakhan, Rey. "Canada's Health System: Charting a New Vision for the 21st Century." Paper presented at the conference Health Care: International Comparisons. King's College, London, Eng., 7 July 1994.

Parker, Jr., Shafer. "Tomorrow Never Comes." *BC Report* 8 June 1998: 10–12.

Parsons, Arthur, and Patricia Parsons. *Patient Power! The Smart Patient's Guide to Health Care*. Toronto: U of Toronto P, 1997.

Paul, Alexandra. "Breast Cancer Tests Lagging." *Winnipeg Free Press* 18 Mar. 1998: A1.

Pear, Robert. "States Take Lead in Health Legislation." *New York Times* 14 Sept. 1998: A12.

Pollard, Stephen. "Britain's NHS: Coping with Change." Ramsay, McArthur, and Walker 3–14.

Poplin, Caroline. "Managed Care." *Wilson Quarterly* 20.3 (1996): 15.

Powell, J. Enoch. *Medicine and Politics: 1975 and After*. Tunbridge Wells, Eng.: Pitman Medical Publishing, 1976.

Priest, Lisa. "Condition Critical as Health System Nears 30." *Toronto Star* 23 Sept. 1995: A1.

——. *Operating in the Dark: The Accountability Crisis in Canada's Health Care System*. Toronto: Doubleday, 1998.

Quinn, Mark. "Some Hip Replacement Patients Waiting 3 Years." *Medical Post On-Line* 6 Oct. 1998.

Rachlis, Michael, and Carol Kushner. *Second Opinion: What's Wrong with Canada's Health-Care System and How to Fix It*. Toronto: Collins, 1989.

——. *Strong Medicine: How to Save Canada's Health Care System*. Toronto: HarperCollins, 1994.

Ramsay, Cynthia. "Medical Savings Accounts: Universal, Accessible, Portable, Comprehensive Health Care for Canadians." *Critical Issues Bulletin*. Vancouver: Fraser Institute, 1998.

——. Telephone interview. May 1997, Mar. 1998.

Ramsay, Cynthia, William McArthur, and Michael Walker, eds. *Healthy Incentives: Canadian Health Reform in an International Context*. Vancouver: Fraser Institute, 1996.

Ramsay, Cynthia, and Michael Walker. "A Thriving Health Care Sector Could Contribute to a Healthy Economy." *Fraser Forum* Oct. 1996: 7–21.

——. *Waiting Your Turn: Hospital Waiting Lists in Canada*. Vancouver: Fraser Institute, 1998.

Rees, Matthew. "Defensive Medicine." *Weekly Standard* 2 June 1997: 14.

Reform Party of Canada. *A Fresh Start for Canadians: A 6 Point Plan to Build a Brighter Future Together*. Ottawa: Reform Party of Canada, 1996.

——. "Taxes and Health Care: It's Critical. Pre-Budget Submission of the Official Opposition." Feb. 1999.

Reid, Angus. *Shakedown: How the New Economy Is Changing Our Lives*. Toronto: Seal, 1997.

Richards, John. *Retooling the Welfare State: What's Right, What's Wrong, What's to Be Done*. Toronto: C.D. Howe Institute, 1998.

Robson, Bill. Telephone interview. Feb. 1997.

Roch, D.J., Robert G. Evans, and David Pascoe. "Manitoba and Medicare." *Manitoba Health* Mar. 1985: 21.

Rosenberg, Elliot. Letter to the Editor. *New York Times* 18 Sept. 1991: A18.

"Rx for the Health Care System." *Wall Street Journal* 8 Oct. 1998: A18.

Saskatchewan Health Services Utilization and Research Commission. *Reducing Non-Urgent Use of the Emergency Department: A Review of Strategies and Guide for Future Research*. Regina: SHSURC, 1998.

Saul, John Ralston. Address. The Future of Health Care conference, the Canadian Medical Association, Ottawa, 26 Feb. 1999.

Sillars, Les. "Red Alert in the Legislature: Politicians Wince as Alberta Hospitals Struggle with Another Apparent Spike in Demand." *Alberta Report* 9 Mar. 1998: 12–13.

Solomon, Lawrence. "Empowerment to the People." *Globe and Mail* 4 July 1998: D9.

Storey, Richard. "Giving the Reforms a Chance." *Patients or Customers: Are the NHS Reforms Working?* Ed. Reginald Murley. London, UK: Institute of Economic Affairs, 1995.

Sullivan, Patrick. "Once More into the Breach as Reform MP-MDs Prepare for a Federal Election." *Canadian Medical Association Journal* 156 (1997): 1315–16.

Thorpe, Kenneth E. "Inside the Black Box of Administrative Costs." *Health Affairs* 11.2 (1992): 41–55.

"Three Die While on Heart Waiting List." *Southam News* 25 Feb. 1997.

Toneguzzi, Mario. "Health Care: Even Canada's Most Fiscally Conservative Politicians Know They Mess with Medicare at Their Peril." *Calgary Herald* 15 Oct. 1993: A5.

Trifunov, David. "A Deadly Waiting Game." *Ottawa Citizen* 5 Mar. 1998: A1.

Ulrich, Volker. "Health Care in Germany: Structure, Expenditure, and Prospects." Ramsay, McArthur, and Walker 63–84.

"United Non-Alternative." *Ottawa Citizen* 3 June 1998: A13.

"Victims of Medicare." *British Columbia Report* 8 June 1998: 10–13.

Waldo, Daniel R., and Sally T. Sonnefeld. "US/Canadian Health Spending: Methods and Assumptions." *Health Affairs* 10.2 (1991): 159–64.

Walker, Michael. "Canadians with Medical Needs Follow Their Doctors South." *Wall Street Journal* 5 Mar. 1999: A15.

——. Letter. *Health Affairs* 11.2 (1992): 233–35.

——. Telephone interview. May 1998.

——. "Why Canada's Health Care System Is No Cure for America's Ills." Washington, DC: Heritage Foundation, 1989.

Walker, Robert. "Alberta Heart Surgery Patients Waiting Too Long: Study." *Medical Post* 11 Nov. 1997: 57.

——. "Waiting Lists Are an Accepted Part of Canadian Health System." *Medical Post* 20 Feb. 1996: 66.

Wallace, James. "Ticket to Nowhere?" *Toronto Sun* 4 Feb. 1998: 2.

Weber, Joseph. "Canada's Health-Care System Isn't a Model Anymore." *Business Week* 31 Aug. 1998: 36.

Weidman, Miriam. Telephone interview. May 1997.

Wickens, Barbara. "Scanners and Blasters." *Maclean's* 15 June 1998: 22.

Williams, J. Ivan, and C. David Naylor. "Patterns of Healthcare in Ontario #5, Hip and Knee Replacement in Ontario." Unpublished essay, Institute for Clinical Evaluative Studies, U of Toronto, 1993.

Wilson, Jim. Address to the Empire Club, Toronto. 26 Apr. 1996.

Wilson-Smith, Anthony. "Reform on a Roll." *Maclean's* 11 Oct. 1993: 17–19.

Winsor, Hugh. "Manning Would End Universal Medicare: Fees or Premiums Called Inevitable." *Globe and Mail* 12 June 1992: A7.

Wysong, Pippa. "Canadian Patients Worse Off?" *Medical Post* 17 Feb. 1997: 1.

Zelder, Martin. Telephone interview. Mar. 1999.